FIX
YOUR INSULIN

7 Simple Hacks to Lose Weight
Without Hunger or Calorie Counting

Burn Fat. Stay Lean—For Good.

KARL JACOB

ISBN: 979-8-9950151-0-9 (paperback)
ISBN: 979-8-9950151-1-6 (e-book)
ISBN: 979-8-9950151-2-3 (audio)

Published by Wellingtonia Publishing LLC

For more information, visit FixYourInsulin.com.

Scan with your phone's camera or visit the link above.

NO COMMERCIAL ENDORSEMENTS STATEMENT

This book contains recommendations for foods, supplements, kitchen tools, and lifestyle practices based solely on the author's personal experience and research.

The author receives no compensation, commission, or financial benefit from any products, brands, or services mentioned in this book. All recommendations are made in good faith to help you achieve your health goals.

You have the freedom to select any brands, products, or alternatives that align with your budget and preferences. Regardless of the specific products you use, the principles in this book remain applicable.

ACKNOWLEDGMENTS

This book is not intended as an academic work and, as such, may contain unintentional instances of plagiarism. The content has been compiled with the intention of sharing knowledge and insights, rather than adhering to strict academic standards or citation practices.

I appreciate your understanding and hope that you find value in the ideas presented here.

MEDICAL DISCLAIMER

The information in this book is for educational and informational purposes only and is not intended as medical advice, diagnosis, or treatment. The author is not a physician, registered dietitian, licensed nutritionist, or healthcare provider.

Before starting any new diet, exercise program, or fasting protocol, or introducing changes to your current health regimen, consult a qualified healthcare professional.

The strategies described in this book may not be appropriate for everyone. You should not attempt the dietary changes or fasting protocols in this book if you:

- Are pregnant or breastfeeding
- Have been diagnosed with or are at risk for eating disorders
- Have type 1 diabetes or take insulin medication
- Have kidney disease, liver disease, or pancreatic conditions
- Have a history of heart disease or take blood pressure medication
- Take any medications that dietary changes might affect.
- Are under 18 years of age
- Have any other medical condition or health concern

If you are currently medicated for diabetes, blood pressure, or any other condition, dietary changes can affect your medication needs.

Work closely with your healthcare provider to monitor your progress and adjust medications as necessary.

Individual results will vary. The author's 80-pound weight loss is his personal experience and does not guarantee results. Sustainable weight loss depends on many factors, including starting weight, metabolism, adherence, medical conditions, genetics, and individual physiology.

If you experience any adverse symptoms while following the advice in this book—including but not limited to dizziness, chest pain, severe fatigue, irregular heartbeat, or any other concerning symptoms—discontinue immediately and seek medical attention.

The author and publisher do not accept responsibility or liability for any consequences resulting directly or indirectly from using this book's information.

By reading and applying the information in this book, you accept full responsibility for your health decisions.

AUTHOR'S NOTE

Over a decade ago, I weighed 280 pounds and received a diagnosis that changed my life: dangerously high insulin levels and a clear path toward type 2 diabetes within a few years.

I was terrified. I had four children, a devoted wife, and a life I desperately wanted to live fully. But I was trapped in a body that was failing me—or so I thought.

What I discovered over the next four years transformed not just my body, but my entire understanding of weight loss, metabolism, and health. I lost 80 pounds. My insulin levels normalized. My energy soared.

And most importantly, I've kept the weight off for over a decade.

But this book isn't just my story. It's a synthesis of scientific research, practical experimentation, and hard-won wisdom about what actually works for sustainable weight loss.

What you won't find in this book:

- Calorie counting or food weighing
- Extreme restriction or deprivation
- Expensive supplements or meal replacement shakes
- Gimmicks, quick fixes, or unrealistic promises

What you will find:

- Seven practical, science-based strategies that address the root cause of weight gain: insulin resistance
- A framework you can implement gradually, one hack at a time
- Flexibility built into the system so you can actually live your life
- Real talk about challenges and setbacks, and advice on how to navigate them

I'm not a doctor or a registered dietitian. But I am someone who struggled with weight for years, tried everything, failed repeatedly, and finally discovered an approach that worked—and kept working.

My goal is straightforward: to share what I've learned so you won't have to spend years struggling as I did.

Your transformation begins now.

With encouragement and belief in your success,

Karl

CONTENTS

HOW TO USE THIS BOOK

This book is structured around 7 simple hacks that work together to address insulin resistance and create sustainable weight loss.

Each hack builds on the others, creating a complete system that transforms how your body processes food, burns fat, and maintains energy.

THE 7 HACKS YOU'LL LEARN:

Hack #1: The Food Order Secret

Hack #2: Low-Glycemic Swaps That Satisfy

Hack #3: Intermittent Fasting Made Easy

Hack #4: Turn Your Life Into a Fitness Routine

Hack #5: Healthy Fats and The Ketosis Secret

Hack #6: The Science Behind Meal Prep and Real Food

Hack #7: The 80/20 Flexibility Principle

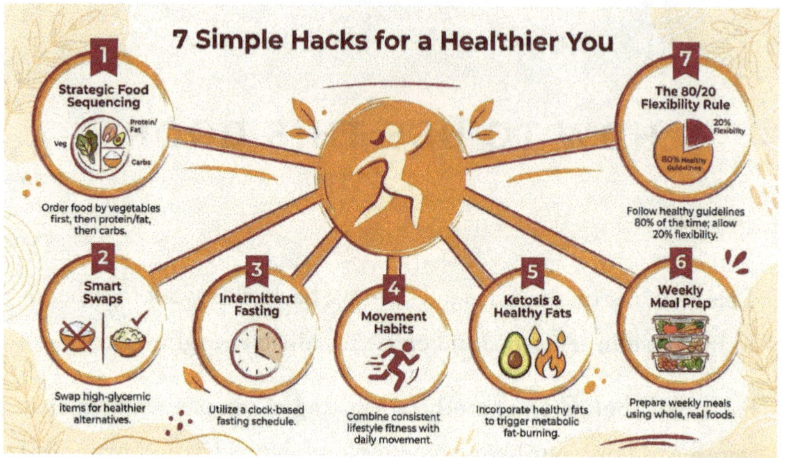

These seven strategies are built on these five foundational principles:

H – Hormone Balance (understanding insulin's role)

A – Adaptive Eating (food order, meal timing, intermittent fasting)

C – Carb Awareness (low-glycemic swaps and strategic carb intake)

K – Ketosis Benefits (leveraging fat-burning metabolism)

S – Sustainable Habits (meal prep, movement, flexibility)

Hack Your Health: The H.A.C.K.S. Framework

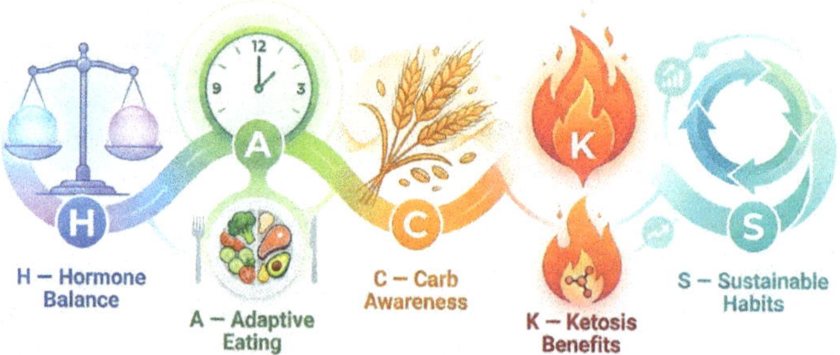

Together, they form a complete framework for metabolic health and lasting weight loss.

TWO APPROACHES TO IMPLEMENTATION:

OPTION 1: The Gradual Build (Recommended for Most People)

Implement one hack per week to allow your body and mind to adapt gradually.

- Week 1: Start with Hack #1 (Food Order)—eat vegetables first at every meal
- Week 2: Add Hack #2 (Low-Glycemic Swaps)—make three strategic food swaps
- Week 3: Introduce Hack #3 (Intermittent Fasting)—begin with 12:12 schedule
- Week 4: Add Hack #4 (Movement)—implement the seven-minute morning routine
- Week 5: Explore Hack #5 (Healthy Fats and Ketosis)—if it aligns with your goals
- Week 6: Establish Hack #6 (The Science Behind Meal Prep and Real Food)—craft a weekly meal prep routine
- Week 7: Integrate Hack #7 (80/20 Flexibility)—for sustainable long-term balance

By Week 8, all 7 hacks are working together as a complete system.

OPTION 2: The All-In Approach (For Highly Motivated Individuals)

If you're ready to dive in completely, you can implement all 7 hacks simultaneously. Be prepared for:

- A more intense initial transition (especially in weeks 1-2)
- Potential "keto flu" symptoms if entering ketosis rapidly
- Faster initial results
- Higher likelihood of needing to adjust and fine-tune as you go

Note: Even with the all-in approach, I recommend reading the entire book first to understand how all the pieces fit together.

HOW THE BOOK IS ORGANIZED:

Chapters 1-2: Foundation (why diets fail, how insulin works, your starting point)

Chapters 3-9: The 7 Hacks (one chapter per hack, with detailed implementation)

Chapter 10: Maintenance (sustaining results for life, troubleshooting challenges)

Chapter 11: Beyond Weight Loss (the more profound transformation you'll experience)

SPECIAL FEATURES IN EACH HACK CHAPTER:

The Science Behind It—Understanding Why It Works

My Personal Story—How I discovered and applied this hack

Step-by-Step Implementation—Exactly how to do it

Common Mistakes to Avoid—Pitfalls I acquired this knowledge through difficult experiences.

Quick-Win Challenge – A practical action step to implement this week

A FINAL NOTE BEFORE YOU BEGIN:

This isn't about perfection. It's about progress.

You'll have wonderful days and challenges. You'll implement some hacks easily and struggle with others. You might lose weight quickly at first, then hit plateaus. You might slip up at social events or under stress.

All of this is normal. All of this is part of the journey.

What matters is that you keep showing up. Keep implementing. Keep learning from your body's feedback.

Your transformation doesn't happen in a moment—it unfolds over time through consistent action.

📥 CLAIM YOUR FREE BONUSES

As a thank you for purchasing this book, I've created two free resources to help you put the 7 Hacks into action:

🎁 THE HABIT SCORECARD

Want to gamify your transformation? I've created The Fix Your Insulin Habit Scorecard—an eight-week tracking system that turns the 7 Hacks into a daily game. Score yourself, build streaks, and watch your progress stack up. To learn each hack, read the book first, then get your scorecard to apply it and build lasting habits.

🎁 THE SCIENCE DEEP-DIVE GUIDE

All 64 peer-reviewed references are organized by topic, with key takeaways summarized.

Download both free at:
FixYourInsulin.com/bonus

Scan with your phone's camera or visit the link above.

You're ready. Let's begin.

CHAPTER 1

MY 280-POUND WAKE-UP CALL

The paper gown crinkled with every nervous shift I made on the examination table in Dr. Martinez's office. Fluorescent lights hummed overhead, casting that particular shade of clinical white that makes everything feel sterile and final. The smell of antiseptic mixed with faint coffee from the break room down the hall. It was a typical Tuesday morning for everyone but me.

I was 48 years old, 6 feet 3 inches tall, and weighed 280 pounds. But honestly? I felt fine. Great, even. I had energy for my work, I was managing four kids with my devoted wife, and life was ... busy. Chaotic. But fine.

That's why I was completely taken aback when Dr. Martinez entered, clutching my lab results and displaying an expression that made my stomach sink.

He sat down slowly, the way doctors do when they're about to change your life.

"Your blood pressure looks good," he began, and I started to relax. "Heart rate is normal."

Then, he delivered a devastating statement: "Your insulin levels are dangerously high." And they're climbing."

I stared at him, confused. Insulin? I'd heard of it, vaguely. It had to do with diabetes. Wasn't that something that happened to other people? People who were ... well, sicker than me?

"If this trend continues," he said, his voice measured and serious, "you're looking at Type 2 Diabetes within three to five years. Maybe sooner. And once you're on that path... medication, potential complications, nerve damage, cardiovascular disease..." He trailed off, allowing the implications to hang in the air.

The words blurred together. My mind went to my four children—their laughter, needs, and futures. I thought of my wife, the foundation of our family, who had supported me through everything. I wondered about my future: Would I live to see my kids graduate? Get married? Have kids of their own?

For the first time in my life, I understood what real fear felt like.

Understanding What My Body Was Telling Me

After giving me my results, Dr. Martinez could see the confusion on my face. He leaned forward, and what he said next would become the foundation of everything I'd learn over the next four years.

"Let me explain what insulin resistance actually means. Your body produces insulin to move glucose—sugar—from your bloodstream into your cells for energy. But when you eat too many carbohydrates, especially refined ones, your body has to produce more and more insulin to do the same job. Eventually, your cells stop responding well to insulin. They become 'resistant.'"

He drew a simple diagram on his notepad. "Think of it like this: insulin is the key that unlocks your cells to let glucose in. But with insulin resistance, it's like the locks are rusty. You need more and more keys—more insulin—to get the same result. Meanwhile, all that excess insulin is telling your body to store fat and never let it go."

He paused, and his tone shifted to something I desperately needed to hear: *hope*.

"Here's the critical part: Type 2 diabetes and insulin resistance can often be reversible with lifestyle changes. Unlike Type 1 diabetes, which is an autoimmune condition where the pancreas can't produce insulin, Type 2 is often driven by lifestyle factors. That means you may be empowered to change this."

That word—reversible—hit me like lightning.

This was not necessarily a sentence of life. This was a wake-up call. And I might be empowered to answer it.

The Silent Warning Signs I'd Been Ignoring

Looking back now, the warning signs were everywhere. I didn't know how to identify them.

Dr. Martinez handed me a printout and started explaining the warning signs of insulin resistance and pre-diabetes. As he spoke, I realized with growing alarm that I'd been experiencing nearly all of them. I'd just dismissed them as usual—part of getting older, being busy, and being a dad.

Here's what I'd been ignoring:

1. Constant Cravings (Especially for Carbs and Sugar)

I couldn't get through an afternoon without hitting the vending machine. Cookies, chips, candy bars, you name it. I always told myself I "deserved a treat" after a hard day. But the truth was, I *needed* them. The cravings were relentless, and I'd built my entire eating schedule around feeding them.

What was really happening: My blood sugar was spiking and crashing repeatedly, triggering intense biological signals for a quick energy boost. It wasn't weakness—it was metabolic dysfunction.

2. Energy Crashes Two to Three Hours After Meals

Every day, precisely at 2 p.m., I would experience a breakdown. I'd feel exhausted, foggy, and irritable. I'd reach for coffee, sugar, or anything to push through. I thought it was just part of life—everyone feels worn out after lunch.

What was really happening: My blood sugar was spiking dramatically after meals, triggering massive insulin release, then crashing below normal levels. This glucose roller coaster was draining my energy and focus.

3. The "Apple-Shaped" Body (Belly Fat)

I carried most of my weight around my midsection. My arms and legs were relatively standard, but my belly was where most of my weight settled. That's where everything settled. I joked about my "beer belly" and bought bigger pants.

What was really happening: Visceral belly fat—the kind that accumulates around your organs—is one of the most concerning types. It's often a sign that insulin is working too well at its storage function, packing fat exactly where it can be most metabolically problematic.

4. Brain Fog and Difficulty Concentrating

I'd sit at my desk, struggling to focus. Simple tasks felt overwhelming. I chalked it up to stress, being a parent of four, and work pressure. However, it seemed as though my brain was functioning through a dense mist.

What was really happening: My brain wasn't getting steady fuel. Blood sugar spikes and crashes were disrupting my brain, preventing it from reaching the stable glucose levels necessary for optimal cognitive function.

5. Feeling Tired Even After Sleeping

Even after sleeping for seven or eight hours a night, I would wake up feeling as if a truck had struck me. No amount of rest seemed to help. I started wondering if something was seriously wrong with me.

What was really happening: My body was working overtime at the cellular level to manage chronically elevated blood sugar and insulin. I was exhausted not from lack of sleep but from metabolic stress that never stopped.

6. Darkened Skin Patches (Neck, Armpits)

I noticed some darkening on the back of my neck and in my armpits. I thought it was dirt, poor hygiene, or maybe even aging. I'd scrub at it in the shower, frustrated that it wouldn't come off.

What was really happening: This condition, called acanthosis nigricans, is often a visible sign of insulin resistance. My body was literally showing me—on the outside—what was happening inside.

7. Frequent Urination and Thirst

I was always thirsty. Always. And I was constantly running to the bathroom. I thought maybe I was drinking too much water or that my bladder was weak.

What was really happening: My body was trying to flush out excess glucose through my urine. The constant thirst was my body's way of replacing the fluids I was losing.

8. The Big One: Feeling "Fine" While the Numbers Climbed

This was the most dangerous sign of all. Despite everything I just described, I genuinely felt fine. I thought I was doing great. And that's precisely why insulin resistance is sometimes called a "silent" condition. You don't always feel it creeping up on you until it's significantly advanced.

Are You Insulin Resistant? 8 Warning Signs to Watch For

A simple visual checklist of common but often overlooked symptoms indicating potential insulin resistance.

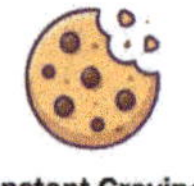

Constant Cravings
Often for sugary or high-carb foods.

Energy Crashes
Especially after meals.

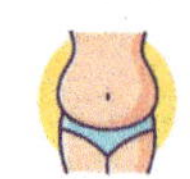

"Apple-Shaped" Body
Signified by excess belly fat.

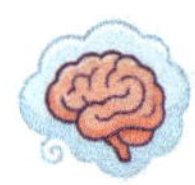

Brain Fog
Difficulty concentrating or remembering things.

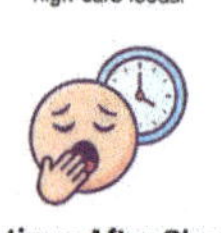

Fatigue After Sleep
Waking up feeling tired.

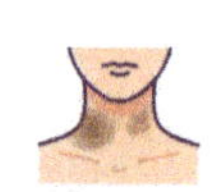

Darkened Skin Patches
Often on the neck or armpits.

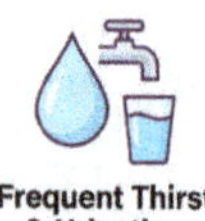

Frequent Thirst & Urination
A classic sign of blood sugar issues.

Feeling 'Fine'
The most dangerous sign is ignoring subtle symptoms.

What was really happening: My body was compensating, adapting, and working harder and harder to maintain some semblance of normal function. But it couldn't keep it up forever.

Dr. Martinez looked at me across the desk and said, "Your body is screaming at you. You just haven't learned its language yet."

That day, I started learning.

The Night Everything Changed

I drove home from that appointment in silence, Dr. Martinez's words echoing in my head. *Three to five years. Diabetes. Medication. Complications.*

That evening, I stood in the soft light of my living room, listening to my children's laughter echoing through the house. They were playing some game, joyful and utterly unaware of the storm churning inside me. My wife was in the kitchen, the familiar sounds of dinner preparation a comforting rhythm I'd taken for granted for too many years.

But I couldn't shake Dr. Martinez's face. The lab results. The timeline.

I felt the weight of the world on my shoulders. I'd let my work consume me. I'd prioritized everything except my own health. And now? Now I was facing the very real possibility of not being there for the people I loved most.

The tears came suddenly, hot and unbidden. I wasn't a crier—I was the guy who held it together, who solved problems, and who kept moving forward. But in that moment, something broke open inside me.

How could I face my children knowing I'd let myself become this person? How could I look into my wife's eyes—the woman who had stood by me through everything—when I'd become a shadow of the man she'd married?

My heart ached with the thought of their disappointment. I imagined my kids growing up without their father. I imagined missing graduations, weddings, and grandchildren, all because I'd ignored the warning signs. All because I thought I was "fine."

But standing there in that moment, surrounded by the laughter and love that made my life worth living, I made a vow:

I would not let my family suffer because of my ignorance. I would not let the life we'd built together slip away. I would fight—for them, for the laughter that filled our home, for the love that had always been our foundation.

That night became my turning point.

I would reclaim my life not just for myself but for them.

The Decision: I Had a Choice (And You Have One, Too)

In that moment, I understood something fundamental: I had a choice.

I could ignore Dr. Martinez's warning, the way I'd ignored all the other signs. I could keep living the way I'd been living, hoping things would magically improve. I could wait until the diagnosis became official, until the medications started, until the complications became unavoidable.

Or I could take control. Right now.

I chose the latter.

But here's the thing—and this is important for you to understand: I'd tried dieting before—multiple times. And every single time, I'd failed.

I'd count calories religiously, starve myself, lose a few pounds, and then gain it all back—plus more. It was the classic yo-yo effect that millions of people experience, trapped in an endless cycle of hope and disappointment. I'd feel hungry all the time, miserable, and deprived. And eventually, I'd give up.

So I knew that whatever I did this time had to be different. I couldn't rely on willpower alone. I couldn't just "eat less and move more." That hadn't worked before, and it wasn't going to work now.

I needed to understand what was actually happening in my body. I needed to learn the language my body had been speaking all along— the language of insulin.

Discovering the Insulin Connection

For weeks after that appointment, I dove deep into research. I read everything I could find about insulin, insulin resistance, blood sugar, metabolism, and fat storage. I watched lectures, read studies, and talked to doctors and nutritionists.

And slowly a picture began to emerge—a picture that explained *everything.*

Every failed diet. Every moment of seemingly unstoppable hunger. Every pound I'd regained after swearing, "This time would be different."

It wasn't my fault. It wasn't a lack of willpower. It wasn't some character flaw or moral failure.

It was insulin.

My body wasn't broken. It was responding exactly as evolution designed it to respond. When I ate carbohydrates—especially the refined, processed carbs I'd been living on—my blood sugar spiked. My pancreas responded by releasing insulin into my bloodstream. And that insulin did precisely what it was designed to do: help store energy for later.

The problem was that, with insulin resistance, my cells weren't appropriately responding to insulin's signals. So my pancreas kept producing more and more, desperately trying to clear the glucose from my blood. And all that excess insulin kept signaling my body: "Store fat! Don't burn it! We might need it later!"

As long as my insulin levels remained consistently high, I was effectively locked out of my own fat reserves. It didn't matter how few calories I consumed or how much I exercised. My body couldn't efficiently access its stored fat for energy because my insulin system wasn't functioning correctly.

This was the missing piece I'd been searching for my entire adult life.

And once I understood that, everything changed.

Instead of fighting my body, I could work *with* it. Instead of forcing myself into starvation and misery, I could address the root cause. Instead of another failed diet, I could achieve actual, lasting transformation.

The 7 Hacks That Saved My Life

Over the next four years, I lost 80 pounds. My insulin levels normalized. My energy soared. My brain fog disappeared. I stopped craving sugar. I stopped feeling hungry all the time. And most importantly, I stayed there. I didn't put the weight back on.

I didn't do it through deprivation, calorie counting, or misery. I did it by understanding my body's insulin response and working with it, not against it.

I discovered seven simple strategies—hacks that made weight loss feel effortless, sustainable, and even enjoyable. These weren't complicated protocols that required a PhD in nutrition to understand. They were practical, actionable changes I could implement immediately and see results within days.

Here's a preview of the 7 hacks you'll learn in this book:

Hack #1: The Food Order Secret—Eat your vegetables first, your protein and fats second, and your carbohydrates last. Research suggests this simple change can potentially reduce your post-meal glucose spike by up to 73 percent.

Hack #2: Low-Glycemic Swaps That Satisfy—Learn which foods spike your insulin and which keep it stable. It's not about eating less; it's about eating smarter.

Hack #3: Intermittent Fasting Made Easy—Give your body the metabolic rest it may desperately need. I started experimenting with intermittent fasting back in 2012, long before it became mainstream. It changed everything for me.

Hack #4: Turn Your Life Into a Fitness Routine—You don't need a gym membership or hours of cardio. From my seven-minute morning Tabata protocol to turning housework into exercise, movement can become effortless when you incorporate it into your daily life.

Hack #5: Healthy Fats and The Ketosis Secret—Once my body learned to burn fat for fuel instead of sugar, my cravings vanished entirely.

Hack #6: The Science Behind Meal Prep and Real Food—If it has more than five ingredients, it's not real food. Meal prep, shopping strategies, and cooking have become my secret weapons.

Hack #7: The 80/20 Flexibility Principle—Rigid perfection leads to failure. Sustainable flexibility leads to lasting success. This hack is what makes everything else sustainable for life.

An Important Note About Your Journey

Before you begin, I need to be honest with you: your journey may look different from mine.

You might lose weight faster than I did. You might lose it more slowly. You might lose 20, 50, or 100 pounds. Your results will depend on many factors: your starting weight, your metabolism, how closely you follow the strategies, your stress levels, your sleep quality, your hormonal health, your genetics, and dozens of other variables I can't predict.

There are no guarantees with weight loss. Anyone claiming otherwise isn't honest.

But if you implement these strategies consistently, research suggests your body will likely respond. Your insulin levels may improve. Your energy may increase. Your cravings may diminish. Your health markers may get better.

And for most people who follow these principles, weight loss does occur. Maybe not 80 pounds. Maybe not in four years. But progress happens.

The question isn't whether these strategies can work. The question is, will you work for them?

Will you show up every day, even when it's hard? Will you keep going when you hit plateaus? Will you learn from your mistakes and adjust? Will you trust the process even when results feel slow?

If you can answer yes to those questions, then I'm confident your transformation is possible.

Not immediate. Not always easy. But possible.

What This Book Will Do for You

This book isn't a diet. It's not a temporary fix or a quick gimmick. It's a blueprint for understanding your body's language and working with it to achieve sustainable, lasting weight loss.

If you've thoroughly explored all options without success, please know that it is not your fault.

The diet industry has been misleading people for decades. They've told you that weight loss is just about calories in versus calories out. They've told you to eat less and move more. They've made you feel like a failure when their flawed advice didn't work.

But the truth is, your body is more complex than a simple math equation. And once you understand the role of insulin—one of the master hormones that influences fat storage—you'll finally have a key to unlocking sustainable weight loss.

Over the following few chapters, I'm going to walk you through exactly what I did. I'll explain the science in simple, accessible terms (no PhD required). I'll share my personal experiences, my struggles, and my breakthroughs. And most importantly, I'll give you the exact hacks I used to lose 80 pounds and keep them off.

This isn't just about weight loss. It's about reclaiming your life. It's about waking up with energy, playing with your kids without getting winded, looking in the mirror, and feeling proud. It's about potentially improving the health markers that concern you and living with vitality and strength.

This is about becoming the person you were always meant to be.

Your Journey Starts Now

Fixing my Insulin changed my life. Throughout this book, I will demonstrate how it can transform your life.

Let's do this together.

Welcome to your transformation.

But before we dive into the 7 hacks, you need to understand why every diet you've tried has failed—and why this time will be different. That's what we'll explore in Chapter 2.

CHAPTER 2

WHY YOUR DIET KEEPS FAILING (AND WHY FIXING YOUR INSULIN CHANGES EVERYTHING)

If you've ever lost weight only to gain it all back—plus a few extra pounds for good measure—you're not alone. In fact, you're part of the majority.

Studies show that approximately 80 to 95 percent of people who lose weight through traditional dieting regain it within one to five years. That's not a small failure rate. That's nearly everyone.

So let me ask you something: if almost everyone fails at traditional dieting, is the problem really you? Or is it possible that the entire approach is fundamentally flawed?

I'm here to tell you it's the latter. And once you understand why, you'll never look at weight loss the same way again.

The Calorie Myth That's Been Holding You Back

For decades, we've been sold a simple equation: Calories In vs. Calories Out.

The logic seems bulletproof: If you eat fewer calories than you burn, you'll lose weight. If you eat more calories than you burn, you'll gain weight. Simple math, right?

Except your body isn't a calculator. It's a complex biological system governed by hormones, not arithmetic.

Here's what the "calories in, calories out" model gets wrong: it treats all calories as equal. It assumes that 100 calories of broccoli has the same effect on your body as 100 calories of candy. It ignores the hormonal signals that food sends to your body—signals that determine whether you store fat or burn it. That is the calorie deficit trap.

Let me share a real-world example from my life—one that changed everything for me.

My 1,800-Calorie Nightmare

When I was at my heaviest—280 pounds and facing that terrifying diagnosis from Dr. Martinez—I did what every desperate person does: I turned to calorie counting.

I downloaded every popular app. I bought a food scale. I weighed and measured everything I put in my mouth. Chicken breast: 165 calories. Steamed broccoli: 55 calories. Brown rice: 215 calories. I became obsessed with the numbers.

I calculated my Total Daily Energy Expenditure (TDEE) using online calculators. For a 280-pound, 6'3" man with moderate activity, it came out to roughly 3,200 calories per day to maintain my weight. So I created what seemed like a massive deficit: I ate only 1,800 calories per day.

That's a 1,400-calorie deficit. According to the conventional wisdom that "3,500 calories equals one pound of fat," I should have been losing nearly 3 pounds per week.

The first two weeks? It worked. I lost 8 pounds. I felt victorious. I thought, "Finally! This is working! I just needed to be more disciplined!"

I posted about it on social media. I told my wife, "I've figured it out this time." I bought smaller clothes in anticipation.

Then, week three hit.

The scale didn't move. Not a single pound.

I double-checked my tracking. I weighed everything even more carefully. I made sure I wasn't missing any "hidden" calories. Everything was accounted for. Still 1,800 calories per day. Still a massive deficit.

Week four: Still nothing.

Week five: Still nothing.

I was starving and constantly thinking about food. Irritable. Exhausted. My workouts felt impossible; I had no energy. I'd lie in bed at night, my stomach growling, fantasizing about pizza and ice cream.

I felt like a failure. Again.

So I did what the fitness forums and diet books told me to do: I cut my calories even further down to 1,500 per day.

The result?

I *gained* two pounds.

I stared at the scale in disbelief. How was this possible? I was eating less than half of what I supposedly needed to maintain my weight, exercising regularly, doing everything "right"—and I was gaining weight.

That's when something inside me broke. Not my resolve, but my belief in the system.

I remember sitting at my kitchen table, food scale in front of me, tracking app open on my phone, and thinking, "This doesn't make sense. Something is fundamentally wrong here."

I was exhausted. Hungry. Miserable. And heavier than when I'd started the extreme restriction.

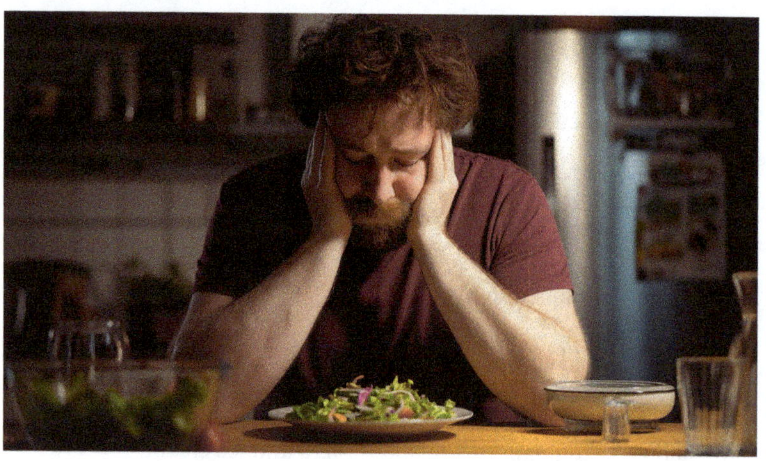

That moment of despair became my breakthrough.

I stopped asking, "What am I doing wrong?" and started asking, "What if the entire approach is wrong?"

That question led me down a path of research that would eventually save my life. But first, I needed to understand what my body was actually doing in response to my calorie restriction.

Why Your Body Sabotages Your Diet

When you drastically cut calories—as I did—your body doesn't say, "Great! Let's burn some fat!"

Instead, it says, "Uh oh. We're starving. Better to slow everything down and conserve energy."

This is called metabolic adaptation, and it's a survival mechanism hardwired into your DNA over millions of years of evolution. Your body doesn't realize you're trying to fit into the jeans you wore in college. It perceives a famine and does everything possible to keep you alive.

Here's what happens when you severely restrict calories:

1. Your Metabolism Slows Down

Your body reduces its energy expenditure to match your reduced calorie intake. You burn fewer calories at rest. You feel more tired. You move less without even realizing it. Your body is literally trying to conserve every calorie it can.

Research has shown that people who lose weight through severe calorie restriction can experience a metabolic slowdown of 20 to 30 percent. That means if you were burning 2,000 calories a day before your diet, you might only be burning 1,400 to 1,600 after several weeks of restriction—even if your activity level stays the same.

My experience: That 3,200-calorie TDEE I calculated? After five weeks of restriction, my body had probably adapted down to around 2,200–2,400. So my 1,800-calorie intake wasn't creating the deficit I thought it was. My body had altered the rules that applied to me.

2. Your Hunger Hormones Go Haywire

When you restrict calories, your body increases production of ghrelin—the "hunger hormone." Ghrelin is like your body's alarm system, screaming, "Feed me! We're starving!"

At the same time, your body decreases leptin—the "satiety hormone" that tells you when you're full. So you're hungrier than ever, and nothing satisfies you.

This is why willpower alone doesn't work. You're not weak. You're fighting against powerful biological signals that evolved over millions of years to keep you alive during times of scarcity.

My experience: I couldn't stop thinking about food. I'd dream about it. I'd watch cooking shows to vicariously experience eating. Every social gathering became torture. The mental obsession was as exhausting as physical hunger.

3. You Lose Muscle, Not Just Fat

When you create a severe calorie deficit without properly managing your hormones, your body doesn't just burn fat. It also breaks down muscle tissue for energy.

This is catastrophic for weight loss, because muscle is a metabolically active tissue. In fact, modern science now recognizes muscle as an organ—one of the most important organs for our metabolism. The more muscle you have, the more calories you burn at rest. When you lose muscle, your metabolism slows even further.

My experience: I got smaller, but I also got weaker. My body looked "soft"—what people call "skinny fat. "I'd lost weight, but I hadn't transformed my body. And my metabolism was now even more damaged than before.

4. Your Body Becomes a Fat-Storage Machine

Here's the cruelest irony of all: severe calorie restriction can actually make you *better* at storing fat.

When your body experiences prolonged calorie deprivation, it becomes more efficient at extracting every possible calorie from food and storing it as fat—just in case another "famine" is coming.

So when you finally give up on your restrictive diet (and you will, because it's unsustainable), your body pounces on every calorie and stores it away. This is why so many people end up heavier than when they started.

My experience: When I eventually gave up on the 1,500-calorie restriction, I gained back the eight pounds I'd lost plus five more. I was now 13 pounds heavier than when I'd started my "successful" diet.

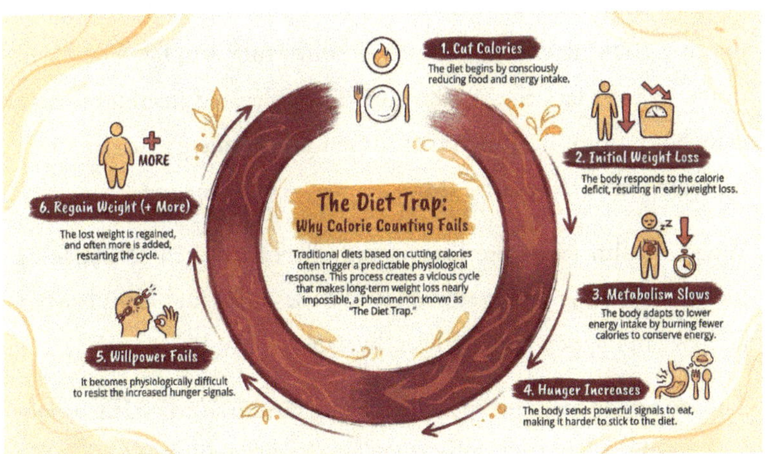

It's not your fault. It's biology.

The Real Culprit

Calorie counting doesn't work long-term.

The answer lies in understanding and managing insulin—a master hormone that plays a crucial role in fat storage and fat burning.

Let me explain how insulin actually works, because this is the key to everything.

Insulin: Your Body's Metabolic Switch

Your pancreas produces insulin in response to rising blood sugar. Its primary job is to move excess glucose (sugar) out of your bloodstream and into your cells, where it can be used for energy.

But insulin has another critical function that most people don't understand: it acts as a master switch, determining whether your body stores energy or burns it.

When insulin levels are elevated, your body is in "storage mode." It prioritizes taking excess glucose and converting it to fat, which gets stored in your fat cells. At the same time, elevated insulin prevents your body from breaking down stored fat for energy. It essentially prevents access to your fat stores.

When insulin levels are low, your body can switch to "burning mode." It gains access to stored fat and uses it for fuel. This is when fat loss can happen more efficiently.

This switching mechanism is what makes insulin so crucial for weight loss. Insulin has a direct impact on your body's ability to reach its fat stores, unlike a straightforward calorie arithmetic. You can eat in a calorie deficit, but your body may find it difficult to properly burn stored fat if your insulin levels are consistently high.

Similar to how a vault door opens and valuable energy escapes, lower insulin levels allow the body to access and use its stored fat as fuel. Just as the state of the vault door controls whether energy is stored or released, insulin levels determine whether the body may access its fat reserves.

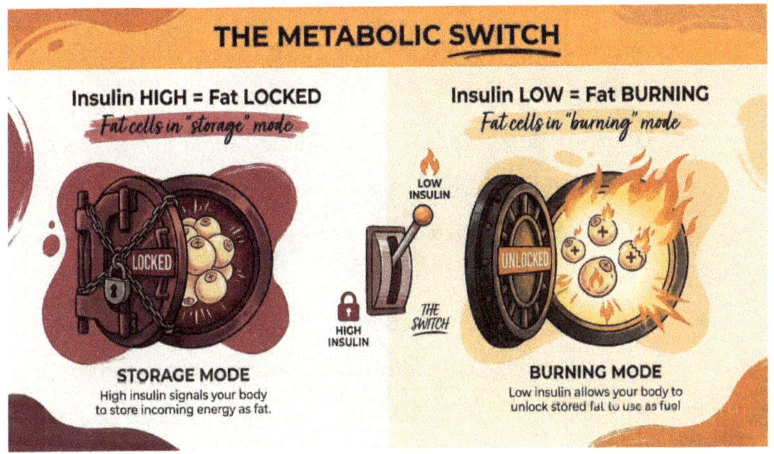

This is why *what* you eat determines your insulin response far more than *how much* you eat.

Not All Calories Are Equal

Let me give you two scenarios to illustrate this critical point:

Scenario A: High-Carb Breakfast

You eat a bowl of sugary cereal with low-fat milk and a glass of orange juice—total calories: approximately 400.

What typically happens:

- The moment the food hits your mouth, your blood sugar begins to rise rapidly.
- Your pancreas releases a surge of insulin to handle the glucose flood.
- The insulin drives glucose into your cells and signals the conversion of excess glucose to fat.
- Insulin remains elevated as long as it's needed to process the glucose.
- As insulin does its job and drives blood sugar down, you can end up in a low blood sugar state—sometimes even lower than where you started. This triggers intense cravings: „We need more sugar NOW!"
- Two hours later, your blood sugar crashes. You feel hungry and tired, and you are desperately craving more carbs.
- Your body stays in fat-storage mode all morning.
- The cycle repeats at lunch.

Scenario B: Low-Carb, High-Fat Breakfast

You eat scrambled eggs cooked in butter with avocado slices and a side of spinach—total calories: approximately 400.

What typically happens:

- Your blood sugar rises minimally.
- Your pancreas releases a small amount of insulin.
- The fat and protein provide steady, sustained energy.
- Four to five hours later, you're still satisfied.
- Your insulin levels stay low, allowing for potential fat-burning.

- Your body can remain in fat-burning mode all morning.
- No cravings, no crashes.

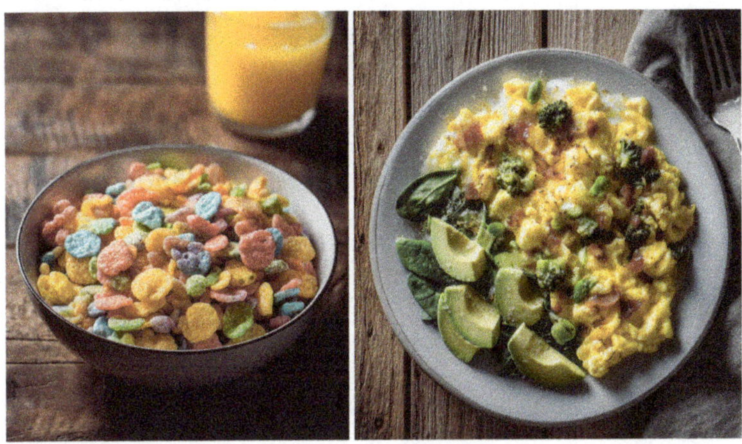

Same calories. Completely different hormonal response. Completely different outcome.

This is why I could eat 1,800 calories of the "right" foods and potentially lose weight effectively, while 1,800 calories of the "wrong" foods left me hungry, worn out, and stuck on a plateau.

The quality of your calories matters more than the quantity.

Now, I want to be clear: this doesn't mean you can eat unlimited amounts of high-quality food without consequences. Even nutrient-dense foods can contribute to weight gain if consumed in excess. However, this rarely becomes a problem because foods high in healthy fats, protein, and fiber have powerful satiating qualities. They fill you up and keep you satisfied far longer than processed carbs ever could.

This is where the concept of volumetrics becomes essential. High-quality, whole foods tend to be lower in calorie density but higher in volume and nutrients. They physically fill your stomach and trigger natural fullness signals. But you still need to listen to your body carefully and stop eating once you feel satisfied, not stuffed. Pay attention to genuine hunger versus habit, boredom, or emotional eating.

The H.A.C.K.S. Framework and The 7 Hacks

Now that you understand why traditional dieting fails and how insulin works, let me introduce you to the framework that will guide your transformation.

This isn't just a collection of random tips. It's a comprehensive system for managing your insulin, optimizing your metabolism, and achieving sustainable weight loss.

I call it The H.A.C.K.S. Framework—five core principles that underpin everything you'll learn in this book:

H – Hormone Balance

A – Adaptive Eating

C – Carb Awareness

K – Ketosis Benefits

S – Sustainable Habits

These five principles work together to address the root cause of weight gain: insulin resistance. But principles alone aren't enough— you need practical strategies to put them into action.

Over the following seven chapters (Chapters 3-9), I'll share 7 specific, actionable strategies—the 7 Hacks—that apply these principles in your daily life. Each hack is practical, immediately implementable, and scientifically proven to work.

Think of the 5 H.A.C.K.S. principles as the foundation—the why behind everything you'll do. Think of the 7 Hacks as the house you'll build on that foundation—the *what* you'll actually implement. The principles explain why insulin matters and how your body works. The hacks give you specific strategies to put those principles into practice. Together, they create a complete system for lasting transformation.

Here's how the framework and the hacks connect:

THE H.A.C.K.S. FRAMEWORK (5 Core Principles)

H – Hormone Balance

Master your insulin response by understanding which foods spike it and which keep it stable. Learn to work with your body's hormonal signals—insulin, ghrelin, and leptin—instead of fighting against them.

This isn't about perfection; it's about awareness. Once you understand how different foods affect your hormones, you can make informed choices that support your goals rather than sabotage them.

Applied in: Hacks #1, #2, and #5

A – Adaptive Eating

Implement strategies like food order (vegetables first, carbs last), intermittent fasting, and meal timing to optimize your body's fat-burning potential. This isn't about restriction—it's about intelligent adaptation.

When you constantly bombard your body with insulin-spiking foods without rest, it struggles to keep up. But when you give it the right inputs at the correct times, it responds beautifully.

Applied in: Hacks #1, #3, and #6

C – Carb Awareness

Understand the quality and timing of carbohydrates. Not all carbs are problematic, but quality, quantity, and timing matter enormously. Learn which carbs serve your goals and which work against them.

This isn't about eliminating carbs forever. It's about being strategic—choosing carbs that provide nutrition without triggering metabolic chaos.

Applied in: Hacks #2 and #7

K – Ketosis Benefits

Learn how to shift your body from burning sugar to burning fat through nutritional ketosis. This is optional but powerful—and it's one of the secrets to eliminating cravings once and for all.

Ketosis isn't required for weight loss, but understanding it gives you another powerful tool in your arsenal.

Applied in: Hack #5

S – Sustainable Habits

Build practical, enjoyable habits around meal prep, movement, and mindset. Weight loss only works if you can sustain it for life, and sustainability comes from making healthy choices easy and enjoyable.

This is where most diet books fail. They give you the information but don't show you how to integrate it into real life. The H.A.C.K.S. framework is designed for sustainability from day one.

Applied in: Hacks #4, #6, and #7

THE 7 HACKS (Practical Strategies)

These five principles come to life through seven specific strategies you'll learn in the chapters ahead:

Hack #1: The Food Order Secret *(Hormone Balance + Adaptive Eating)*

Eat vegetables first, protein and fats second, and carbs last. This will reduce glucose spikes by up to 73 percent.

Hack #2: Low-Glycemic Swaps That Satisfy *(Hormone Balance + Carb Awareness)*

Simple food substitutions that stabilize insulin without leaving you feeling deprived.

Hack #3: Intermittent Fasting Made Easy *(Adaptive Eating)*

Give your metabolism the rest it needs to unlock fat-burning and autophagy.

Hack #4: Turn Your Life Into a Fitness Routine *(Sustainable Habits)*

From seven-minute morning rituals to turning housework into exercise—movement becomes effortless.

Hack #5: Healthy Fats and The Ketosis Secret *(Hormone Balance + Ketosis Benefits)*

The craving-killer that changed everything for me—learn to burn fat for fuel.

Hack #6: The Science Behind Meal Prep and Real Food *(Adaptive Eating + Sustainable Habits).*

Meal prep, shopping strategies, and cooking become your secret weapons.

Hack #7: The 80/20 Flexibility Principle *(Carb Awareness + Sustainable Habits)*

The key to maintaining your results forever, without perfection or deprivation.

Why This Framework and These Hacks Work Together

This approach is different because:

- ☑ It addresses the root cause (insulin) rather than symptoms (weight).
- ☑ It's flexible enough to adapt to your life, not the other way around.
- ☑ It doesn't require calorie counting or food weighing.
- ☑ It builds on itself—each hack amplifies the others.
- ☑ It's sustainable for life, not just a few months.
- ☑ It's both principle-based and action-oriented—you understand why it works and know exactly what to do.

Over the following seven chapters, I'll walk you through each hack in detail, showing you exactly how to implement it, why it works, and how to avoid the common mistakes I made along the way.

By the end, you'll have both the knowledge and the practical strategies to lose weight without hunger. You'll be able to keep the weight off forever and feel better than you have in years.

The Three Macronutrients: A Quick Overview

Before we dive into the individual hacks, you need a basic understanding of how different types of food affect your body. All food can be broken down into three macronutrients: carbohydrates, proteins, and fats. Each one triggers a different insulin response.

1. Carbohydrates: The Insulin Trigger

Carbohydrates generally have the most significant effect on insulin. When you eat carbs, they're typically broken down into glucose, which enters your bloodstream. Generally, the more refined carbohydrates you consume, the more rapidly your blood sugar can rise, often triggering a stronger insulin response.

However, not all carbs affect your body equally. Some carbs are digested quickly and cause rapid spikes in blood sugar (like white bread, candy, and soda). Others are digested more slowly and cause gentler rises (like vegetables, legumes, and some whole grains).

Fiber content, processing level, and overall nutrient density all influence how quickly carbs raise blood sugar. We'll dive deeper into choosing the right carbs in Chapter 4.

What you need to know now: Refined, processed carbohydrates are typically your biggest insulin challenge. Whole food sources with fiber tend to have a gentler impact.

2. Protein: The Moderate Impact

Protein has a modest effect on insulin compared to carbohydrates. Your body does release some insulin in response to protein, but it's typically a much gentler, more controlled response.

Protein also has some unique benefits:

- It's highly satiating, keeping you full for hours.
- It supports muscle growth and repair.
- It requires more energy to digest (higher thermic effect).
- It stimulates hormones that signal fullness.

However, too much protein can be counterproductive. When you eat excessive amounts of protein, your body can convert the excess into glucose through a process called gluconeogenesis. This can raise blood sugar and insulin levels, potentially hindering fat loss.

The sweet spot for most people is a moderate protein intake—roughly 20 to 30 percent of your daily calories, or about 0.8 to 1.2 grams of protein per kilogram of body weight.

3. Fats: Minimal Insulin Impact

Interestingly, healthy fats have minimal impact on insulin levels compared to carbohydrates.

When you eat fat, your blood sugar doesn't spike significantly. Your pancreas doesn't need to release large amounts of insulin. Your body can stay in a more neutral metabolic state.

This is why fat became my secret weapon for weight loss. Not only did it keep me satisfied for hours, but it also allowed my body to maintain lower insulin levels, which meant better access to stored fat for energy.

There is an important distinction, though—not all fats should be treated equally.

Fats to Prioritize (healthy fats):

- Avocados and avocado oil
- Olive oil (extra virgin)
- Fatty fish (salmon, mackerel, sardines)
- Nuts and seeds (almonds, walnuts, chia seeds, flaxseeds)
- Coconut oil and MCT oil
- Grass-fed butter or ghee

Fats to Minimize:

- Trans fats (hydrogenated oils in processed foods)
- Highly processed vegetable oils (excessive amounts of soybean, corn, and canola)
- Anything deep-fried in low-quality oils

We'll explore fats in much more detail in Chapter 7, including how to use them strategically for fat loss and overall health.

Your Choice: Stay Stuck or Move Forward

You're standing at a crossroads right now.

You can go back to what you've always done—counting calories, fighting hunger, and hoping this time will be different while using the same broken strategies.

Or you can embrace a new approach based on science, experience, and results. A strategy that works with your body instead of against it.

I chose the second path while sitting in Dr. Martinez's office, staring at those terrifying lab results. And it saved my life.

Now it's your turn.

Fix Your Insulin isn't just about weight loss. It's about reclaiming your energy, your health, your confidence, and your future. It's about being there for the people you love. It's about waking up every morning feeling strong, capable, and in control.

Let's get started with Hack #1. You don't need to count calories or measure portions to start losing weight. You need to change the order in which you eat your food. That's precisely what we'll explore in Chapter 3: Eat Your Vegetables First.

HACK #1—THE FOOD ORDER SECRET

If I told you that you could reduce your blood sugar spike by up to 73 percent simply by changing the *order* in which you eat your food—without eliminating any foods—would you believe me?

I wouldn't have believed it either. It sounds too simple. Too good to be true.

But it's not only true—it's one of the most powerful, immediately actionable strategies for managing insulin and accelerating weight loss. And the best part? You can start using it at your very next meal.

This is Hack #1: The Food Order Secret.

How I Discovered the Power of Food Order

About six months into my weight loss journey, I was already seeing results from cutting back on refined carbs and eating more whole foods. But I was still experiencing occasional blood sugar crashes in the afternoons, and strangely, my weight loss had started to plateau.

One evening, while reading about glucose management strategies, I came across a study that completely halted my progress. In research published in the *European Journal of Clinical Nutrition*, scientists found that when participants ate vegetables before carbohydrates, post-meal glucose spikes were reduced by up to 73 percent compared to eating the same foods in mixed or reverse order.

The same meal. The same calories. Just a different sequence.

I sat there staring at the screen, my mind racing. Could it really be that simple?

The next morning, I decided to test it. Instead of my usual breakfast—where I'd eat everything mixed together—I deliberately ate my foods in a specific order:

1. First: A hefty serving of sautéed spinach and mushrooms
2. Second: Scrambled eggs cooked in butter
3. Last: A small portion of sweet potato

Within 30 minutes, I noticed something remarkable: I didn't get that familiar post-breakfast energy dip—no mid-morning cravings for a snack. I felt satisfied, steady, and clear-headed.

I kept experimenting with this approach over the next several weeks, and the results were undeniable. My afternoon crashes disappeared. My cravings diminished. And when I stepped on the scale after a few weeks, I'd broken through the plateau that had frustrated me.

That's when I learned that the order of your food is as important as what you eat.

The Science Behind Food Order

So why does eating vegetables first make such a dramatic difference? The answer lies in how your digestive system processes food and how different foods affect your blood sugar.

The Fiber Speed Bump Effect

When you eat fiber-rich vegetables first, a transformation begins in your digestive tract. Think of fiber as creating a series of speed bumps. When carbohydrates arrive later in the meal, they have to navigate through this fibrous barrier, which slows down how quickly glucose enters your bloodstream. Instead of a rapid flood, you get a gentle, steady release—like a controlled drip instead of a fire hose.

Without this fiber barrier, carbohydrates are absorbed rapidly, causing a sharp blood sugar spike—and the corresponding insulin surge that locks you into fat-storage mode.

The Research That Proves It Works

Multiple studies have confirmed the power of food sequencing:

Study 1: Cornell University (Weill Cornell Medical College)

Researchers found that eating vegetables before carbohydrates reduced post-meal glucose spikes by 73 percent and insulin spikes by 48 percent compared to eating carbohydrates first. Participants ate the same foods—just in a different order.

Study 2: Japanese Research on Food Order

A study published in the *European Journal of Clinical Nutrition* showed that eating vegetables and protein before rice significantly lowered post-meal blood sugar levels in people with type 2 diabetes. The effect was so pronounced that researchers suggested food sequencing as a practical intervention for blood sugar management.

Study 3: The Protein and Fat Buffer

Additional research has shown that eating protein and fat before carbohydrates further slows gastric emptying—the rate at which food leaves your stomach. The slower your stomach empties, the more gradually glucose enters your bloodstream, the smaller your insulin response, and the longer you feel satisfied.

The science is precise: food order matters—a lot.

The Optimal Food Order Strategy

Here's the exact sequence I use at every meal, and it's the same sequence I recommend you start implementing today:

The Food Order Secret: Hack Your Meals for Better Health

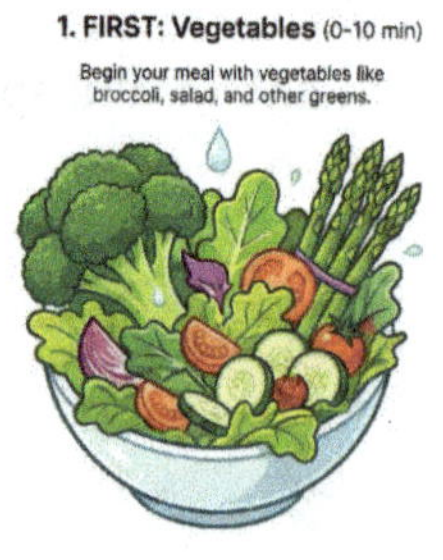

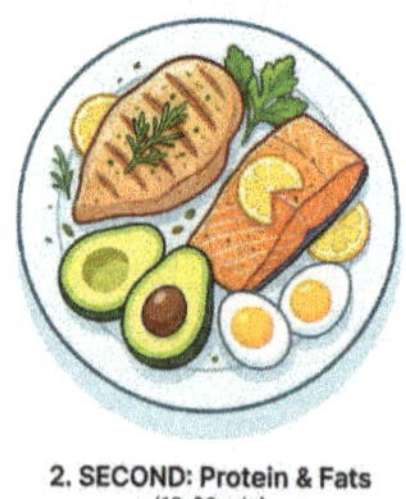

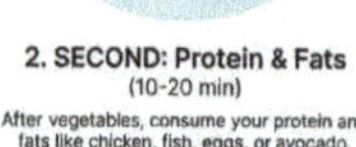

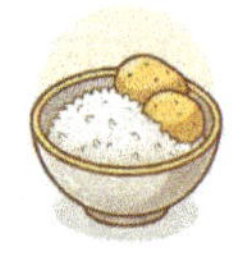

Step 1: Vegetables First (10 Minutes)

Start every meal with non-starchy, fiber-rich vegetables. Eat them first, before anything else touches your lips.

Best Choices:

- Leafy greens (spinach, kale, arugula, lettuce)
- Cruciferous vegetables (broccoli, cauliflower, Brussels sprouts, cabbage)
- Zucchini, cucumber, bell peppers, asparagus, green beans
- Mushrooms, celery, radishes

How much?

Fill at least half your plate with vegetables. If you're eating at a restaurant, order a side salad or a vegetable starter and eat it in its entirety before your main course arrives.

Why It Works:

These vegetables are loaded with fiber and water but very low in calories and carbohydrates. They create the speed bump effect in your digestive tract and start triggering satiety signals, so you naturally eat less of the higher-calorie foods that come later.

What this looks like in practice: I'd sit down with my plate and spend the first 10 minutes of every meal eating only the vegetables—maybe two cups of roasted broccoli or a large mixed salad. I'd savor each bite, chew thoroughly, and only after finishing would I move on to the next component. No rushing. No mixing everything.

Step 2: Protein and Healthy Fats Second (10 to 15 Minutes)

After you've finished your vegetables, move on to protein and fats.

Best Choices:

- Protein: Eggs, chicken, turkey, beef, pork, fish, tofu, tempeh
- Healthy Fats: Avocado, olive oil, nuts, seeds, cheese, fatty fish

Why It Works:

Protein and fat further slow digestion and provide sustained energy. They also keep you feeling full, reducing the likelihood that you'll overeat the carbohydrates that come next. Plus, they have a minimal impact on insulin levels, keeping you in fat-burning mode.

What this looks like in practice: After finishing my vegetables, I'd spend another 10 to 15 minutes on the protein portion of my meal—a grilled chicken thigh, a piece of salmon, or scrambled eggs. If there were healthy fats like avocado or nuts, I'd eat those at this point, too.

Step 3: Carbohydrates Last (If at All)

Finally—and only after you've eaten your vegetables, protein, and fat—you can eat your carbohydrates.

Best Choices:

- Sweet potatoes, quinoa, brown rice, wild rice
- Legumes (lentils, chickpeas, black beans)
- Small portions of whole grains or starchy vegetables

How much?

Keep your carb portions modest—roughly the size of your fist or about 1/2 to 1 cup. By the time you've eaten your vegetables and protein, you'll likely find that you're already quite satisfied and don't need as much as you might expect.

Why It Works:

By eating carbs last, they encounter the fiber barrier and the slowed digestion from protein and fat. This dramatically reduces the glucose and insulin spike. In many cases, I found that I didn't even want or need the carbs by the time I got to this stage—I was already full and satisfied.

A Note on Flexibility:

If you have digestive issues, diabetes, or take medications that affect blood sugar, consult your healthcare provider before making significant changes to your eating pattern. While food order is generally safe and beneficial for most people, individual responses can vary. Listen to your body and adjust as needed.

Real-World Examples: Food Order in Action

Let me show you how this plays out in real meals:

Example 1: Dinner at Home

Traditional Order (Old Way):

I used to eat my chicken, rice, and broccoli together or in random bites. Blood sugar would spike, I'd feel tired an hour later, and I'd be hungry again by bedtime.

Food Order Strategy (New Way):

1. First (10 minutes): Eat the entire serving of steamed broccoli with a drizzle of olive oil and lemon. Just the broccoli. Nothing else.
2. Second (10 minutes): Eat the grilled chicken thigh with a pat of butter. Take your time. Chew thoroughly.
3. Last (optional): Eat a small portion of brown rice, if you're still hungry. Often, I'd skip this entirely because I was already satisfied.

Result: Steady energy, no cravings, slept like a baby.

Example 2: Restaurant Meal

Traditional Order (Old Way):

The bread basket would arrive, and I'd mindlessly eat two or three rolls before my meal even showed up. When the main course arrived, I'd eat pasta mixed with vegetables and protein. Then, when the dessert menu got passed around, I'd feel compelled to order something sweet.

Food Order Strategy (New Way):

1. Skip the bread basket or ask the server not to bring it.
2. Order a side salad or vegetable appetizer. Eat it entirely before the main course arrives.
3. When the main course arrives, eat all the vegetables on the plate first, then the protein, then the starch.
4. By dessert time, I'm satisfied and have no cravings for sweets.

Result: Felt in control and energized and had no regrets.

Example 3: Fast Food (When There's No Other Option)

Important disclaimer: The best strategy is to avoid fast food entirely. These meals are typically highly processed, loaded with unhealthy fats, sodium, and hidden sugars, and offer minimal nutritional value. However, if you find yourself in a situation where fast food is the only option, at least you can use food-order principles to minimize metabolic damage.

Traditional Order (Old Way):

Order a burger with fries and soda. Eat randomly—fries, burger bites, more fries. Blood sugar spikes wildly. Feel terrible an hour later.

Food Order Strategy (If You Must):

1. First: Order a side salad if available and eat it completely (ask for olive oil and vinegar if possible, or use minimal dressing—most dressings are loaded with sugar).
2. Second: Eat the burger patty and any vegetables/toppings (lettuce, tomato, onion), leaving the bun aside or for last.
3. Last: Have a few fries if you're still hungry (but honestly, you probably won't be).
4. Skip the soda entirely. Order water or unsweetened iced tea instead.

If you have even 10 minutes, rather than eating fast food, find a grocery store and grab pre-made options like a rotisserie chicken, pre-cut vegetables, hard-boiled eggs, or a bagged salad. These are almost always a better choice than fast food.

Result: Better blood sugar control even in suboptimal situations, though still far from ideal.

My Personal Experience: The Transformation

When I first started implementing food order, I was skeptical. It felt almost too easy—like I was getting away with something.

But within the first few weeks, I noticed changes:

- No more afternoon energy crashes.
- Reduced cravings for sweets after meals.
- Smaller portions have led to greater satisfaction.
- This naturally led to a decrease in food portions, as I felt full before completing my plate.
- Ability to go four to five hours between meals without feeling hungry.

The changes grew over the next few months:

- My blood sugar remained stable throughout the day.
- Friends and family started asking what I was doing differently.
- Food order had become completely automatic.
- Restaurants became easy: "I'll start with a salad, please."
- My relationship with carbs had fundamentally changed—they were no longer the star of my meals.

Important Note About My Weight Loss Pattern:

As I mentioned in my overall strategy, I didn't lose weight in a straight line. I would use intermittent fasting (Hack #3) intensively for about a week every four to five weeks, lose several pounds, and then maintain that new weight for the next four to five weeks while eating normally (but while still using food order and the other hacks). This plateau approach allowed my body to adjust to each new weight, reset my metabolic set point, and made the weight loss sustainable. Food order was crucial during those maintenance weeks—it kept my blood sugar stable and prevented weight regain.

The most remarkable part? I wasn't restricting anything. I was still eating the foods I enjoyed. I just ate them in a different order. And that simple change had a profound effect on my insulin levels, my hunger, and my weight.

Common Mistakes to Avoid

As simple as this hack is, there are a few pitfalls to watch out for:

Mistake #1: Eating Everything Mixed Together

If you toss your salad with pasta or stir your vegetables into your rice, you lose the protective effect of the fiber barrier. The foods need to be eaten in sequence, with vegetables coming first.

Solution: Keep foods separate on your plate and eat them in order, one at a time.

Mistake #2: Not Eating Enough Vegetables

A few token pieces of lettuce won't create the fiber barrier you need. You need a substantial serving—at least half your plate—to get the full benefit.

Solution: Make vegetables the most significant component of your meal. Go for volume.

Mistake #3: Rushing Through Your Meal

Eating too quickly doesn't give your digestive system time to respond appropriately. You also miss the satiety signals that tell you when you're full.

Solution: Take at least 10 minutes to eat your vegetables, then another 10 minutes for your protein and fat. Chew slowly. Put your cutlery down between bites. Be present with your food.

Mistake #4: Starting with Carbs

If you eat carbs first—even healthy carbs like fruit or whole grains—you've already triggered an insulin response before the fiber barrier is in place.

Solution: Always start with non-starchy vegetables. Save everything else for later.

Mistake #5: Drinking Sugary Beverages with Your Meal

Soda, juice, sweet tea, or even sweetened coffee can spike your blood sugar instantly, negating the benefits of the food order.

Solution: Stick to water, unsweetened tea, black coffee, or sparkling water with lemon. Water is always the best choice.

Mistake #6: Not Drinking Enough Water

Proper hydration helps digestion and can enhance the feeling of fullness. Many people mistake thirst for hunger.

Solution: Drink a glass of water 20 to 30 minutes before your meal, and sip throughout your meal. This helps fill your stomach and supports the fiber's effectiveness.

Practical Tips for Success

Here are some strategies that helped me make food order a permanent habit:

1. Prep Vegetables in Advance

Every Sunday, I'd wash and chop vegetables for the week—bell peppers, cucumbers, celery, cherry tomatoes, and broccoli florets. Having them ready to go made it easy to start every meal with vegetables.

Store vegetables in clear containers at eye level in your fridge. What you see first is what you'll eat first.

2. Use a Salad as Your "Appetizer"

At home or in restaurants, I began treating salads as non-negotiable appetizers. I'd eat the entire salad—with olive oil and vinegar, never sugary dressing—before the main course.

This became such a habit that now I feel weird if a meal doesn't start with vegetables. My body actually craves them first.

3. Reframe Carbs as a "Dessert."

I started thinking of carbs as a treat that comes at the end of the meal, if I still want them. Often, I didn't. This mental shift made it easier to prioritize vegetables and protein.

You're not eliminating carbs—you're just changing when you eat them. And that timing makes all the difference.

4. Visual Cue: The Plate Method

When building my plate, I'd use this simple visual:

- 50 percent vegetables (non-starchy)
- 25 percent protein and fat
- 25 percent carbs (or less)

I'd eat in that exact order, finishing each section before moving to the next.

5. Explain It to Friends and Family

When eating with others, I'd briefly explain what I was doing: "I'm eating my veggies first—it helps with blood sugar and energy." Most people were curious and supportive. Some even started doing it themselves.

You don't need to preach or make a big deal about it. Just do it naturally, and if someone asks, share briefly.

The Ripple Effect: Beyond Blood Sugar

What surprised me most about food order wasn't just the impact on blood sugar—it was the ripple effect it had on every other aspect of my health and eating habits.

1. Portion Control Became Automatic

Because I was filling up on low-calorie, nutrient-dense vegetables first, I naturally ate smaller portions of the higher-calorie foods. I didn't have to think about it or use willpower—my body didn't want as much.

2. Cravings Disappeared

Stable blood sugar means stable energy and mood. When my blood sugar wasn't crashing, I wasn't desperately craving quick-fix carbs and sugar.

3. Digestion Improved

Eating slowly and deliberately, starting with vegetables, significantly improved my digestion. I experienced less bloating, less discomfort, and more regular bowel movements.

4. I Developed a Healthier Relationship with Food

The food order forced me to slow down and be mindful. I started actually tasting my food, enjoying it, and respecting the signals my body was sending me. Meals became an experience, not just fuel.

5. It Worked in Any Situation

Whether I was at home, at a restaurant, at a party, or traveling, I could always apply food order principles. It gave me a sense of control and confidence, no matter where I was.

Troubleshooting Common Food Order Challenges

Let me address some concerns you might have:

"I don't have time for multiple courses at every meal."

You don't need formal courses. Just eat the components of your plate in order. Vegetables first, protein second, carbs last. Same plate, different sequence. Even spending just five minutes on vegetables before moving to the rest of your meal makes a significant difference.

"My family thinks I'm weird eating this way."

You can explain it: "I read that eating veggies first helps with digestion and energy." Most people respect health choices. Or do it quietly without drawing attention. Often, your family won't even notice—they're focused on their own plates.

"What if I'm at a buffet or potluck?"

Fill your first plate with only vegetables and proteins. Eat that completely. Then, if you're still hungry, go back for small portions of starches. This approach prevents the overwhelm of having everything in front of you at once.

"I keep forgetting to do it."

Use visual cues—place your vegetables at the front of your plate, closest to you. They're literally the first thing you see and reach for. Or put a small sticky note on your dining table for the first week as a reminder: "Veggies first!"

"What about smoothies or mixed dishes like stir-fries?"

For smoothies, you can still apply the principle by drinking a vegetable-heavy green smoothie first, then a protein smoothie. For mixed dishes like stir-fries, try to eat the vegetables and protein first, then the rice or noodles. It's not perfect, but it's better than nothing.

Quick-Win Challenge: Your First Week

For a quick win this week, try the following challenge.

The Seven-Day Food Order Experiment

Day 1-2: Awareness

Just observe how you currently eat. Do you eat everything mixed together? Do you start with carbs? Notice your energy levels and cravings after meals. Keep a simple journal: How do you feel one hour after eating? Three hours after?

Day 3-4: Implementation

Start practicing food order at every meal:

1. Vegetables first (at least half your plate)
2. Protein and fat second
3. Carbs last (if at all)

Don't worry about being perfect. Just try it and notice what happens.

Day 5-7: Optimization

Fine-tune the approach. Notice which vegetables you enjoy most. Experiment with timing. Track how you feel. What changes are you noticing? More energy? Fewer cravings? Better mood?

At the End of the Week:

- How's your energy?
- Have your cravings changed?
- Do you feel more satisfied after meals?
- Have you noticed any weight loss?

Most people see noticeable changes within just a few days. Some see results after their very first meal.

Seven-Day Tracking Chart

Use this simple tracking method:

Day	1	2	3	4	5	6	7
Breakfast ✓							
Lunch ✓							
Dinner ✓							
How I Felt							

Check the box when you successfully eat vegetables first at that meal. Note your energy, mood, and cravings in the "How I Felt" column.

Why This Hack Is So Powerful

Food order is powerful because it's

- ☑ Immediate. You can start right away at your next meal.
- ☑ Simple. No calorie counting, no elimination. Just sequencing.
- ☑ Universal. Works with any cuisine or dietary preference.
- ☑ Sustainable. Easy to maintain for life.
- ☑ Science-backed. Research suggests it can reduce glucose and insulin spikes by up to 73 percent.
- ☑ Foundational. Sets you up for success with all the other hacks.
- ☑ Free. No special equipment, supplements, or programs needed.

When I look back at my 80-pound weight-loss journey, food order was one of the first strategies that made everything else easier. It gave me quick wins, built my confidence, and taught me to work *with* my body's biology instead of against it.

What's Next?

Food order is just the beginning. You've learned how to eat your current foods in a way that minimizes insulin spikes and maximizes fat-burning, but what if you could also *swap* some of those foods for even better alternatives? What if you could eat foods that taste just as good—maybe even better—but have a fraction of the impact on your blood sugar?

That's precisely what you'll discover in the next chapter: Hack #2: Low-Glycemic Swaps That Satisfy.

CHAPTER 4

HACK #2—LOW-GLYCEMIC SWAPS THAT SATISFY

One of the biggest myths about weight loss is that you have to give up all the foods you love.

Pizza? Gone. Pasta? Forbidden. Rice? Off-limits forever.

No wonder so many diets fail. Who wants to live a life of deprivation and sacrifice?

Here's the truth: You don't have to eliminate all your favorite foods. You need to make smarter swaps.

This is Hack #2: Low-Glycemic Swaps That Satisfy—simple substitutions that keep your insulin stable, your taste buds happy, and your weight loss on track.

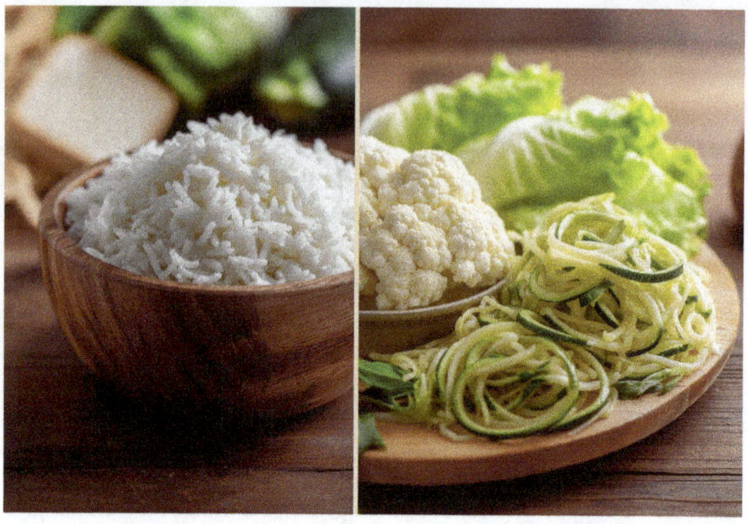

How I Discovered the Power of Smart Swaps

About three months into my weight loss journey, I was seeing solid progress with food order and cutting back on refined carbs. But I'll be honest—I was starting to feel deprived.

I missed pasta. I missed rice. I missed the comfort of a hearty meal that filled me up without making me feel like I was "on a diet."

One Saturday afternoon, I was at the grocery store, wandering the produce section, when I spotted something that caught my eye: pre-riced cauliflower. I'd heard about cauliflower rice before but dismissed it as some trendy diet gimmick that couldn't possibly taste good.

But I was desperate for variety, so I grabbed a bag.

That night, I made my usual stir-fry—chicken, vegetables, and plenty of healthy fats. But instead of white rice, I sautéed the cauliflower rice in a bit of butter and garlic.

I took my first bite, skeptical.

And you know what? It was delicious. Not "good for diet food," but delicious—actually delicious. The texture was different from rice, sure, but it soaked up the stir-fry's flavors beautifully. It was satisfying, filling, and—here's the kicker—I felt great afterward. No blood sugar crash. No food coma. Just steady, sustained energy.

A few weeks later, I discovered another game-changer: shirataki rice and noodles, also known as konjac rice and noodles. Made from the konjac plant root, these alternatives to pasta or rice have almost zero calories and are incredibly beneficial for gut health. The konjac root contains glucomannan, a type of soluble fiber that acts as a prebiotic, feeding the beneficial bacteria in your gut. This resistant starch passes through your small intestine undigested and ferments in your colon, promoting a healthy gut microbiome, improving digestion, and even supporting immune function.

Shirataki became one of my staples. Unlike regular rice and pasta, which spike blood sugar dramatically, shirataki has virtually no impact on insulin levels. Plus, the prebiotic fiber helps you feel fuller longer and supports overall digestive wellness—a true win-win.

Over the next few weeks, I experimented with more swaps—zucchini noodles instead of pasta. Lettuce wraps instead of tortillas. Mashed cauliflower instead of mashed potatoes. Each swap opened up new possibilities, and suddenly, my meals felt abundant and satisfying again.

I didn't need to eliminate foods. I just needed to find better versions. My weight loss accelerated, my energy stayed consistent, and I never felt like I was missing out.

The Science Behind Low-Glycemic Swaps

So why does choosing low-glycemic carbohydrates make such a dramatic difference? The answer lies in how different carbohydrates are structured at the molecular level and how your body processes them.

The Molecular Structure Matters

Not all carbohydrates are created equal. Think of high-glycemic carbs like white bread or white rice as straightforward chains that your body can break down almost instantly—like tearing through tissue paper. Low-glycemic carbs like sweet potatoes or quinoa are more like tightly woven fabric—your digestive system has to work much harder and longer to break them down.

This structural difference changes everything. High-glycemic foods flood your bloodstream with glucose within minutes, triggering a massive insulin spike. Low-glycemic foods release glucose gradually over hours, keeping insulin levels steady and preventing the fat-storage signal.

Without this gradual release, your blood sugar spikes rapidly, insulin surges to compensate, and you're locked into fat-storage mode— followed by an energy crash and intense cravings two to three hours later.

The Research That Proves It Works

Multiple studies have confirmed the power of choosing low-glycemic foods:

Study 1: The Original Glycemic Index Research

Dr. David Jenkins at the University of Toronto pioneered glycemic index research in 1981, demonstrating that different carbohydrates have dramatically different effects on blood sugar—even when they contain the same number of calories. His landmark study in the *American Journal of Clinical Nutrition* showed that white bread spikes blood sugar twice as much as kidney beans, despite both being carbohydrates. This groundbreaking work revealed that not all carbs are created equal.

Study 2: Low-Glycemic Diets and Disease Prevention

A comprehensive review published in *JAMA* by Dr. David Ludwig examined the physiological mechanisms linking glycemic index to obesity, diabetes, and cardiovascular disease. The research showed that high-glycemic foods trigger excessive insulin secretion, promote fat storage, and increase hunger. At the same time, low-glycemic alternatives improve insulin sensitivity, reduce inflammation, and support sustainable weight loss. The study concluded that glycemic index is a critical factor in metabolic health, not just calorie content.

Study 3: The Cochrane Review—Gold Standard Evidence

A rigorous meta-analysis of multiple randomized controlled trials, published in the *Cochrane Database of Systematic Reviews*, examined the effects of low-glycemic diets on diabetes management. The results were compelling: participants following low-glycemic eating patterns showed significantly improved blood sugar control, better A1C levels, and reduced medication requirements compared to standard dietary approaches. The researchers concluded that low-glycemic eating is an effective, evidence-based, practical intervention for metabolic health.

Study 4: Real-World Application

Research compiled in *The New Glucose Revolution* by Jennie Brand-Miller and colleagues demonstrated that simple low-glycemic swaps—like choosing sweet potatoes over white potatoes or quinoa over white rice—can reduce post-meal insulin spikes by 30 to 50 percent without requiring calorie restriction or portion control. These studies showed that small, practical swaps can lead to significant metabolic improvements.

The science is precise: choosing low-glycemic foods stabilizes blood sugar, reduces insulin secretion, and makes weight loss easier.

Understanding Glycemic Load in Real Life

Before we dive into specific swaps, let's quickly review why they work—and introduce a critical concept that will guide all your food choices from now on.

You've probably heard of the Glycemic Index (GI)—a scale that measures how quickly a food raises blood sugar. But there's a more critical measure you need to know about: Glycemic Load (GL).

Glycemic Index (GI): The Incomplete Picture

The Glycemic Index measures how quickly a food raises blood sugar on a scale of 0 to 100, but it doesn't account for portion size or the carbohydrate content of a typical serving. GI only tells you *how fast* a food raises blood sugar, not *how much* it raises blood sugar in a real-world serving.

Example: Watermelon

- GI: 72 (HIGH)
- Sounds terrible. But wait…

Glycemic Load (GL): The Complete Picture

Glycemic Load takes the Glycemic Index and multiplies it by the carbohydrate content of a typical serving, then divides by 100. This gives you a much more accurate picture of how a food will actually affect your blood sugar.

The same example: Watermelon

- GI: 72 (HIGH)
- GL: 4 (LOW)
- Why? Because watermelon is mostly water. A typical serving (about 120 g or 1 cup) only contains about 6 grams of carbohydrate.

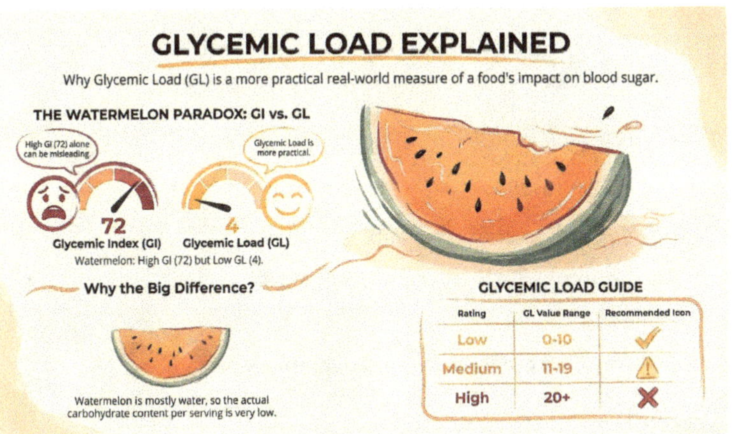

Glycemic Load Categories:

- Low GL (10 or less): Minimal blood sugar impact—your best friends for weight loss
- Medium GL (11 to 19): Moderate impact—fine occasionally, but not daily staples
- High GL (20+): Major blood sugar spikes—these trigger significant insulin surges.

Real-World Comparisons

Let me show you why GL matters more than GI.

Comparison 1: White Rice vs. Cauliflower Rice

White Rice:

- GI: 73 (high)
- GL: 23 (high)
- Typical serving: one cup cooked
- Verdict: Major insulin spike

Cauliflower Rice:

- GI: 15 (low)
- GL: 2 (low)
- Typical serving: one cup
- Verdict: Minimal insulin impact—perfect swap

Comparison 2: Regular Pasta vs. Zucchini Noodles

Regular Pasta:

- GI: 49 (medium)
- GL: 23 (high)

- Typical serving: one cup cooked
- Verdict: Seems moderate, but high GL means a significant insulin response

Zucchini Noodles:

- GI: 15 (low)
- GL: 2 (low)
- Typical serving: one cup
- Verdict: Virtually no insulin impact

Same volume. Same satisfaction. Completely different metabolic impact.

The Takeaway

Focus on Glycemic Load, not just Glycemic Index. When you're evaluating foods, ask yourself, "How much will this typical serving actually raise my blood sugar?"

Low-glycemic swaps are powerful because they let you eat similar volumes and enjoy similar experiences—but with dramatically lower insulin responses.

The Top 12 Low-Glycemic Swaps That Changed My Life

Here are the swaps I relied on most during my 80-pound weight loss journey. These aren't just "tolerable"—they're genuinely delicious and have become permanent fixtures in my diet.

Swap #1: Cauliflower Rice for White Rice

Cauliflower rice has a lower impact on blood sugar than white rice, yet it provides the same texture and "bulk." It's perfect for stir-fries, burrito bowls, and as a side dish. Plus, it's a vegetable—which means it fits perfectly into Hack #1 (eating vegetables first)!

The numbers:

- White rice: GL 23 (high)
- Cauliflower rice: GL 2 (low)

How to prepare:

Buy pre-riced cauliflower (easiest), or pulse cauliflower florets in a food processor until rice-sized. Sauté in a pan with butter or olive oil, garlic, and salt for five to seven minutes. That's it.

Pro tip:

Season it boldly—cauliflower is a blank canvas. Add curry powder, turmeric (a spice known for supporting metabolic health), or fresh herbs to match whatever you're serving it with.

Swap #2: Shirataki Noodles and Rice for Regular Noodles and Rice

Shirataki noodles and rice (made from konjac root) have almost zero calories and zero net carbs. They're a fantastic option for virtually any pasta or rice dish—not just Asian cuisine. I love shirataki and use both the noodle and rice versions regularly.

The numbers:

- Regular noodles/rice: GL 20 to 25 (high)
- Shirataki: GL 0 (zero impact)

How to prepare (My Method):

Rinse the shirataki thoroughly under cold water to remove the natural odor (this is important!). Then, instead of dry-frying (which many recipes recommend), I add them directly to my warm sauce—whether it's tomato, mushroom, or any pasta sauce. They absorb the flavors beautifully, and it's fast, easy, and delicious. No frying needed.

For instance, I'll make my marinara sauce and, instead of traditional pasta, toss in shirataki noodles or rice, letting them heat through in the sauce for a few minutes. Done.

Pro tip:

If you find the noodles too chewy, try the rice version—it has a softer, less chewy texture that many people prefer.

Swap #3: Zucchini Noodles (Zoodles) for Pasta

Zucchini noodles give you that satisfying twirl-on-a-fork experience without the significant insulin spike of traditional pasta. Plus, they're packed with nutrients and fiber. And again—it's a vegetable, so it fits beautifully into Hack #1 as well.

The numbers:

- Regular pasta: GL 23 (high)
- Zucchini noodles: GL 2 (low)

How to prepare:

Use a spiralizer or buy pre-spiralized zucchini. Sauté lightly in olive oil for two to three minutes. Don't overcook them, or they'll get mushy. Top with your favorite pasta sauce, meatballs, or pesto.

Pro tip:

Salt the zoodles and let them sit for 10 minutes before cooking. Pat them dry. This removes excess water and prevents a soggy dish.

Swap #4: Spaghetti Squash for Pasta

When cooked, spaghetti squash naturally separates into noodle-like strands. It's mild, slightly sweet, and pairs beautifully with marinara or meat sauce.

The numbers:

- Regular pasta: GL 23 (high)
- Spaghetti squash: GL 4 (low)

How to prepare:

Cut the squash in half lengthwise, scoop out the seeds, drizzle with olive oil, and roast cut-side down at 400°F (200°C) for 40 to 45 minutes. Use a fork to scrape out the "noodles."

Pro tip:

Don't overcook—you want the strands to have a slight bite, not be mushy.

Swap #5: Lettuce Wraps for Tortillas or Bread

Crisp, refreshing lettuce wraps provide crunch and hold all your fillings without affecting blood sugar. They're perfect for tacos, burgers, and wraps.

The numbers:

- Flour tortilla: GL 8 to 12 (medium)
- Lettuce wrap: GL 0 (zero impact)

Best choices:

Butter lettuce, iceberg, or romaine leaves work best—they're sturdy and flexible.

How to use:

Fill with ground beef or turkey, grilled chicken, tuna salad, or any protein. Add avocado, salsa, and veggies for a complete meal.

Pro tip:

Use two leaves stacked together for extra sturdiness.

Swap #6: Mashed Cauliflower for Mashed Potatoes

Creamy, buttery mashed cauliflower satisfies that comfort-food craving without the starch overload. Most people can't even tell the difference when it's seasoned well.

The numbers:

- Mashed potatoes: GL 17 (medium-high)
- Mashed cauliflower: GL 3 (low)

How to prepare:

Steam cauliflower florets until very soft. Blend or mash with butter, cream, garlic, salt, and pepper. For extra richness, add cream cheese or Parmesan.

Pro tip:

Make sure the cauliflower is completely soft and well-drained before mashing, or it'll be watery.

Swap #7: Almond Flour or Coconut Flour for White Flour

These low-carb flours let you bake bread, muffins, and pancakes without the blood sugar roller coaster. They're also packed with healthy fats and protein.

The numbers:

- White flour: GL 23+ (high, varies by recipe)
- Almond/coconut flour: GL 3 to 5 (low)

How to use:

Substitute almond flour roughly 1:1 in most recipes. Coconut flour is more absorbent—use about 1/4 the amount and add extra eggs or liquid.

Pro tip:

Almond flour works better for savory dishes; coconut flour has a slight sweetness that's great for baked goods.

Swap #8: Greek Yogurt (Full-Fat, Unsweetened) for Sour Cream

Greek yogurt provides the same tangy creaminess as sour cream but with more protein and beneficial probiotics. Choose full-fat versions to keep you satisfied and support healthy eating habits.

How to use:

Top tacos, chili, or baked potatoes (or better yet, baked cauliflower!), or use in dips.

Pro tip:

Strain it through a cheesecloth for a thicker texture.

Swap #9: Avocado or Mashed Banana for Butter/Oil

Avocado adds healthy fats and creaminess to brownies, cakes, and muffins. Mashed banana works too, though it adds natural sugar—use sparingly.

How to use:

Replace butter or oil 1:1 with mashed avocado in chocolate-based recipes (it hides the color). Use ripe bananas for sweetness and moisture.

Pro tip:

Avocado works best in dark chocolate recipes where the green tint won't show.

Swap #10: Coconut Cream or Almond Milk for Heavy Cream

Lower in carbs than dairy cream, coconut cream adds richness to soups, sauces, and coffee. Unsweetened almond milk works for lighter dishes.

How to use:

Use coconut cream in curries, creamy soups, or whipped as a topping. Use almond milk in smoothies or coffee.

Pro tip:

Refrigerate a can of full-fat coconut milk overnight, then scoop the solid cream from the top for dairy-free whipped cream.

Swap #11: Nuts and Seeds for Croutons

Crunchy, satisfying, and packed with healthy fats and protein, nuts and seeds add texture to salads without the blood sugar spike of bread-based croutons.

Best choices:

Almonds, walnuts, pecans, sunflower seeds, and pumpkin seeds.

How to use:

Toast them lightly in a pan with a bit of salt or spices. Toss on salads or roasted vegetables.

Pro tip:

Make a big batch and store it in an airtight container for easy meal prep.

Swap #12: Dark Chocolate (85 percent+ Cacao) for Milk Chocolate

Dark chocolate with high cacao content has minimal sugar and won't spike your insulin like milk chocolate. Plus, it's rich in antioxidants.

The numbers:

- Milk chocolate: GL 10 to 15 (medium, varies by brand)
- Dark chocolate 85 percent or more: GL 4 to 6 (low)

How to enjoy:

Have one or two squares as a treat after dinner. Let it melt slowly in your mouth.

Pro tip:

It takes a few tries to adjust to the more intense, less sweet taste, but once you do, milk chocolate will taste cloyingly sweet. Your palate adapts.

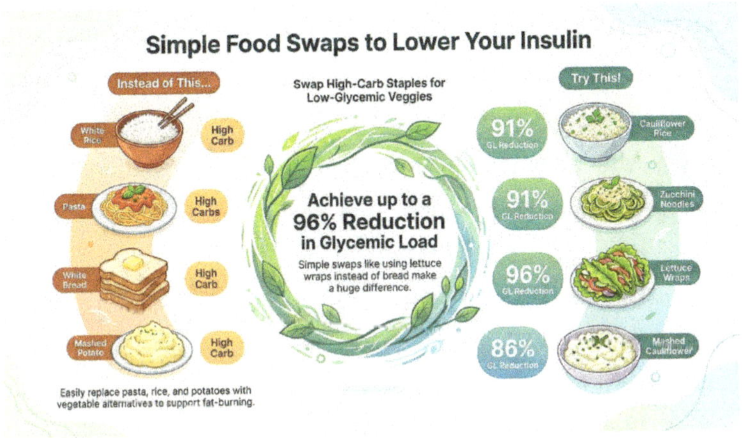

The Five-Ingredient Rule: Real Food vs. Processed Food

Here's one of the most straightforward nutrition rules I ever learned:

If a food has more than five ingredients, it's not real food—it's processed.

Real food is simple. Meat. Fish. Eggs. Vegetables. Nuts. Seeds. Oils. These foods have been nourishing humans for millennia, and they don't need labels or ingredient lists.

Processed food, on the other hand, is designed in a lab to be hyper-palatable, addictive, and profitable. It's usually loaded with hidden sugars, unhealthy fats, preservatives, and chemicals that can wreak havoc on your insulin levels.

How to Apply the Five-Ingredient Rule

Let me show you what this looks like in practice:

- ✅ Chicken breast: one ingredient. Real food.
- ❌ Breaded chicken tenders: Chicken, wheat flour, water, salt, sugar, modified cornstarch, yeast extract, spices, flavor enhancers, preservatives (15+ ingredients). Processed.
- ✅ Almond butter: one ingredient (almonds). Real food.
- ❌ Commercial peanut butter: Peanuts, sugar, hydrogenated oils, salt, artificial flavors, stabilizers (over six ingredients). Processed.
- ✅ Plain Greek yogurt: Milk and live cultures (two ingredients). Real food.
- ❌ Flavored yogurt: Milk, sugar, corn syrup, modified corn starch, artificial flavors, colors, thickeners, and preservatives (10+ ingredients). Processed.

The takeaway: When you stick to real food—foods your great-grandmother would recognize—you naturally avoid the insulin-spiking ingredients that can sabotage weight loss.

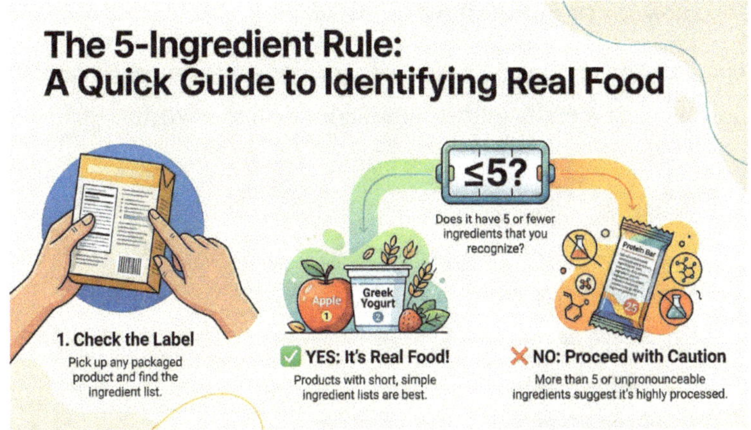

Innovative Shopping Strategies for Low-Glycemic Success

Making low-glycemic swaps starts in the grocery store. Here's how I shop to set myself up for success:

1. Shop the Perimeter

The outer edges of the grocery store are where the real food lives: produce, meat, dairy, and eggs. The inner aisles are where processed foods lurk.

My rule: Spend 80 percent of my shopping time and budget on the perimeter.

2. Read Labels Like a Detective

If a product has more than five ingredients, put it back. If sugar (or its sneaky aliases) appears in the first three ingredients, walk away.

Sugar's Many Disguises: The Complete List

Food manufacturers use dozens of different names for sugar to hide how much is actually in their products. Learn to recognize them all:

Category 1: Syrups

- High fructose corn syrup
- Brown rice syrup
- Agave nectar
- Maple syrup
- Corn syrup
- Malt syrup

Category 2: Words Ending in "-ose" (These are all sugars.)

- Sucrose
- Glucose
- Dextrose
- Fructose
- Maltose
- Lactose

Category 3: Other Disguises

- Maltodextrin
- Evaporated cane juice
- Cane crystals
- Malt extract
- Molasses
- Honey
- Fruit juice concentrate
- Barley malt
- Date sugar

The rule: If any form of sugar appears in the first three ingredients, avoid it. They all spike blood sugar. They're all sugar, just wearing different disguises.

Pro tip: Take a photo of this list on your phone to reference while shopping.

3. Buy in Bulk and Prep Ahead

I buy vegetables in bulk every Sunday and prep them for the week: washing, chopping, and portioning into containers. Having prepped veggies makes healthy eating effortless during busy weekdays.

My weekly prep list:

- Bell peppers, sliced
- Broccoli and cauliflower florets
- Zucchini, spiralized
- Spinach and kale, washed
- Cherry tomatoes, washed

4. Stock Your Pantry with Low-Glycemic Staples

Keep these items on hand so you can always make a healthy meal:

Healthy Fats:

- Olive oil, avocado oil, coconut oil
- Grass-fed butter or ghee

Proteins:

- Canned fish (tuna, salmon, sardines)
- Eggs (always have a dozen on hand)

Nuts and Seeds:

- Almonds, walnuts, macadamia nuts
- Chia seeds, flaxseeds, pumpkin seeds

Dairy Alternatives:

- Coconut milk, unsweetened almond milk

Spices and Flavor:

- Garlic, turmeric, cumin, basil, oregano, cinnamon
- Apple cider vinegar (a secret weapon for blood sugar)

Treats:

- Dark chocolate (85 percent+ cacao)

5. Avoid the „Health Food" Trap

Just because something is labeled "organic," "natural," "gluten-free," or "low-fat" doesn't mean it's good for your blood sugar. Many "health foods" are loaded with hidden sugars.

Examples of deceptive products:

- ❌ Granola bars: Often contain 10-15 g of sugar per bar.
- ❌ Fruit juices: Even "no added sugar" versions spike insulin rapidly (the naturally occurring sugar still affects blood sugar). Water is always the best choice.
- ❌ Low-fat yogurt: Sugar is added to compensate for the loss of flavor.
- ❌ Veggie chips: Often fried and have a similar GL to regular potato chips.
- ❌ "Healthy" cereals: Many contain more sugar than a donut.

Always check the label. Real food doesn't need health claims—it just is healthy.

Budget-Conscious Swaps: Healthy Eating on Any Budget

One of the most significant objections I hear is, "Healthy food is too expensive."

Let me address this directly, because it's simply not true—*if* you shop smart.

Money-Saving Strategies

1. Frozen vegetables are your friend.

They're flash-frozen at peak ripeness, just as nutritious as fresh, and often 50 percent cheaper. I always keep frozen broccoli, cauliflower, and spinach on hand.

2. Buy in-season produce.

I purchase zucchini in the summer, squash in the fall, and Brussels sprouts in the winter. Seasonal = cheaper, fresher, and healthier.

3. Store brands vs. name brands

For basic items (frozen vegetables, canned fish, olive oil), store brands are often identical in quality at 30 to 40 percent lower cost.

4. Bulk buying

Buy items such as nuts, seeds, flours, and oils in bulk from stores like Costco or online. The upfront cost is higher, but the cost per serving drops dramatically.

5. Cook at home

The most significant savings come from eating at home vs. eating out. The cost of one restaurant meal can buy ingredients for three to four home-cooked meals.

Processed food may seem cheaper per item, but when you factor in the long-term health costs—medications, doctor visits, lost productivity—real food is always the better investment.

My Personal Experience: How Swaps Transformed My Diet

When I first started making low-glycemic swaps, I was worried I'd miss the "real" versions of my favorite foods. But something unexpected happened: I stopped wanting the old versions.

After a few weeks of eating cauliflower rice, white rice tasted bland and made me feel sluggish. After enjoying zucchini noodles, regular pasta felt heavy and left me in a food coma. My taste buds adapted, and my body sent clear signals about what made me feel good.

The Cappuccino → Black Coffee Transition

Here's an example from my own journey that shows how changing habits takes time and patience, but it's worthwhile.

I drank a cappuccino every morning, without fail. Then I realized that the milk was triggering my metabolism when I was trying to give my body a metabolic rest during intermittent fasting (more on that in the next chapter). So I switched to black coffee.

At first, it was awful. Bitter. Harsh. I missed the creamy sweetness of my cappuccino.

But I stuck with it. And within two weeks, black coffee started tasting amazing—rich, complex, and energizing. Today, I can't drink cappuccinos anymore. They taste too milky, too sweet, and too heavy.

Your taste buds and preferences absolutely can change. Once you make the shift, you'll wonder why you ever ate any other way.

My Transformation Timeline

Month 1:

- Tried five different swaps
- Found three that I genuinely enjoyed (cauliflower rice, Shirataki noodles and rice, and zoodles)
- Weight loss: eight pounds

Month 2:

- Expanded my repertoire to over ten swaps
- Started experimenting with low-carb baking (almond flour muffins!)
- Meal planning became second nature.
- Weight loss: six pounds (14 total)

Month 3:

- Swaps felt completely normal—not like "diet food."
- Friends and family started asking for my recipes.
- Energy levels are consistently high all day.
- Weight loss: seven pounds (21 total)

Month 6:

- Could go to any restaurant and find low-glycemic options easily
- No longer craved high-carb foods
- Felt in complete control of my diet
- Weight loss: 35 pounds total at this point

The swaps didn't just help me lose weight—they helped me build a sustainable, enjoyable way of eating that I could maintain for life.

Common Mistakes to Avoid with Low-Glycemic Swaps

Even when you're fully committed, setbacks happen. Here are the pitfalls I see most often:

Mistake #1: Giving Up Too Soon

Not every swap will be love at first bite. Give new foods at least three or four tries before deciding you don't like them. Your taste buds need time to adjust.

Try different preparation methods and seasonings. I was hesitant about cauliflower rice the first time because it was too bland. The second time, I added garlic, butter, and lemon zest—total game-changer.

Mistake #2: Overdoing "Keto" Processed Foods

Just because something is labeled "keto" or "low-carb" doesn't mean it's healthy. Many keto products are highly processed and contain artificial sweeteners and unhealthy oils.

Stick to whole, real foods. Make your own versions when possible. Cooking for yourself is how you gain control over your nutrition. There are plenty of easy, fast recipes that don't require much effort to prepare.

Mistake #3: Not Seasoning Enough

Low-glycemic vegetables like cauliflower and zucchini are naturally mild. If you don't season them well, they might taste boring to you.

Be generous with healthy fats (butter, olive oil), salt, garlic, herbs, and spices. Use metabolism-boosting spices such as cayenne, turmeric, cinnamon, ginger, black pepper, cumin, and garlic to enhance both flavor and fat-burning.

Mistake #4: Expecting Exact Replicas

Cauliflower rice isn't white rice. Zoodles aren't pasta. If you go in expecting an identical experience, you'll be disappointed.

Embrace the differences. They're different, and that's okay. Enjoy these foods for what they are—delicious, nutritious alternatives that make you feel amazing. Remember: changing habits takes time and patience, but it's worthwhile.

Mistake #5: Forgetting Portion Control

Just because something is low-glycemic doesn't mean you can eat unlimited amounts. Nuts, cheese, and dark chocolate are all great—but they're calorie-dense.

Pay attention to hunger cues. Stop when you feel satisfied, not stuffed. Practice mindful eating and listen to your body's signals.

Quick-Win Challenge: The Three-Swap Experiment

Choose three swaps from the list above that sound appealing to you. Commit to trying each at least twice this week.

Example Week:

Monday: Cauliflower rice with chicken and vegetable stir-fry (use avocado oil or coconut oil for stir-frying—avoid high-heat vegetable oils)

Wednesday: Shirataki noodles or rice with marinara and meatballs

Friday: Zucchini noodles with mushroom sauce

Track Your Experience:

- For each swap, note:
- How did it taste?
- How did you feel afterward?
- Did it satisfy you?
- Would you make it again?

By the end of the week, you'll likely have two or three new go-to meals that support your weight loss, keep your insulin stable, and taste delicious.

Why This Hack Is So Powerful

Low-glycemic swaps can be powerful because they:

- ☑ Eliminate deprivation. You're not giving up your favorite meals, just upgrading them.
- ☑ May stabilize insulin, resulting in a dramatic reduction in blood sugar spikes.
- ☑ Increase nutrients. Swapping processed carbs for vegetables adds fiber, vitamins, and minerals.
- ☑ Can improve energy—no more post-meal crashes.
- ☑ Support long-term success. These swaps can be sustainable and enjoyable for life.
- ☑ Work anywhere. Home, restaurants, travel—you can always find low-glycemic options.

Low-glycemic swaps were absolutely crucial to my 80-pound transformation. They allowed me to enjoy food, feel satisfied, and stay consistent—all while keeping my insulin in check.

What's Next?

You now know how to swap high-glycemic foods for satisfying low-glycemic alternatives. Your pantry is stocked with wise choices. Your shopping strategy is on point. You understand how to read labels and avoid hidden sugars.

But what if you could give your body extended periods without eating to maximize fat burning and trigger robust cellular repair processes?

That's precisely what we'll explore in Chapter 5: Intermittent Fasting Made Easy.

CHAPTER 5

HACK #3—INTERMITTENT FASTING MADE EASY

In 2012, I accidentally discovered one of the most powerful weight loss strategies I'd ever use—and I did it entirely by accident, years before intermittent fasting became a mainstream phenomenon.

I didn't read about it in a book. I didn't learn it from a guru. I stumbled onto it out of pure necessity, and it changed everything.

This is Hack #3: Intermittent Fasting Made Easy.

If the idea of "fasting" sounds intimidating, restrictive, or impossible, I understand entirely. That's exactly how I felt at first. But intermittent fasting isn't about starving yourself. It's about giving your body strategic periods of metabolic rest so it can access stored fat for energy.

When combined with food order (Hack #1) and low-glycemic swaps (Hack #2), intermittent fasting becomes a force multiplier— accelerating fat loss, eliminating cravings, and making weight management almost effortless.

Let me show you how.

Important: Who Should NOT Fast (Or Who Should Consult a Doctor First)

Before we go any further, I need to be crystal clear about safety. Intermittent fasting isn't appropriate for everyone, so you must decide whether it's right for you.

You should NOT try intermittent fasting if you:

- ✖ Are pregnant or breastfeeding.
- ✖ Have a history of eating disorders (anorexia, bulimia, binge eating disorder).
- ✖ Are under 18 years old.
- ✖ Have Type 1 diabetes or take insulin for Type 2 diabetes.
- ✖ Take medications that must be taken with food.
- ✖ Have a history of hypoglycemia (low blood sugar episodes).
- ✖ Are significantly underweight (BMI under 18.5).
- ✖ Have any chronic medical condition without explicit doctor approval.

You MUST consult your healthcare provider before starting intermittent fasting if you:

- ⚠ Take any prescription medications (timing and absorption may be affected).
- ⚠ Have type 2 diabetes or pre-diabetes (fasting can affect blood sugar significantly).
- ⚠ Have high or low blood pressure.
- ⚠ Have a history of heart problems or irregular heartbeat.
- ⚠ Are over 65 years old.
- ⚠ Have any concerns about how fasting might affect your specific health situation.

Intermittent fasting is powerful precisely because it affects your hormones, blood sugar, and metabolism. That power can be beneficial for many people, but it can also be harmful if you have certain conditions or take certain medications.

Your safety comes first. Always. If you have any doubts about whether intermittent fasting is appropriate for you, talk to your doctor before trying it. Show them this chapter. Get their input.

For everyone else reading this: if at any point during fasting you feel dizzy, extremely weak, confused, or unwell, stop immediately and eat something. Listen to your body. It's always brighter than any book.

Now, with those critical cautions in place, let's explore how intermittent fasting works and why it can be so effective.

My Accidental Discovery of Intermittent Fasting

It was early 2012, about six months into my weight loss journey. I'd already lost about 35 pounds using food order and making low-glycemic swaps, and I was feeling great. But I was still learning, still experimenting, and still paying attention to what my body was telling me.

One evening, after my workout, I felt intensely hungry. It was that familiar, gnawing hunger that made me want to raid the kitchen and eat everything in sight.

But it was late—around 9 or 10 p.m.—and I'd already had dinner hours earlier. I knew eating that close to bedtime wasn't ideal, so I tried to suppress the hunger with a cup of warm herbal tea. I sat there sipping it, hoping it would fill me up and calm the cravings.

It didn't work.

The hunger persisted. My stomach was still growling. I felt unsatisfied, almost irritable.

But I decided: I'm not going to eat. I'm going to bed. I'll have a proper breakfast in the morning.

It wasn't easy. My mind kept wandering to the kitchen, thinking about what I could grab—just something small, to take the edge off. But I stayed strong. I finished my tea, brushed my teeth, and went to bed hungry.

I remember lying there thinking, *This is going to be rough. I'm going to wake up starving.*

But then I fell asleep.

The next morning, something remarkable happened.

I woke up and immediately remembered how hungry I'd been the night before. I braced myself for that same intense hunger to hit me the moment I got out of bed.

But it didn't.

I felt ... fine.

No growling stomach. No desperate need to eat immediately. In fact, I felt surprisingly clearheaded and energized.

I was puzzled. *Wait ... where did the hunger go?*

I made myself a cup of black coffee and waited. I expected the hunger to show up any minute. But it didn't.

Ten a.m. came and went—still nothing.

Eleven a.m. Still fine.

Noon. I felt a slight twinge, but nothing urgent.

It wasn't until around 12 a.m. that I finally felt genuine, physical hunger—the kind that tells you your body actually needs food.

That's when it hit me: my body had fed me.

While I slept, my body had tapped into its own energy stores—my fat reserves—and sustained me through the night and well into the next day. I didn't need external food because my body was burning its internal fuel.

I decided to test it again.

The next evening, I did the same thing. I finished dinner early, had my herbal tea before bed, and went to sleep even though I felt a bit hungry.

The next morning? Same result.

No hunger. Clear mind. Steady energy. And real hunger didn't return until early afternoon.

I repeated this for several days, and the pattern held every single time.

That's when I realized I'd stumbled onto something powerful.

My body wasn't starving. It was thriving. It had switched from burning the food I was constantly feeding it to burning the fat I'd been storing for years. And once that switch flipped, the weight started dropping faster than it ever had with diet changes alone. My energy became rock-solid. My mental clarity was sharper than it had been in years. And most remarkably, my cravings disappeared.

I didn't have a name for what I was doing until months later, when I started researching what was happening in my body. That's when I discovered the term "intermittent fasting" and the science behind its effectiveness.

But it was in that moment, standing in my kitchen at 2 p.m., finally feeling real hunger after over 16 hours without food, when I understood something fundamental: my body didn't need to eat constantly. It just needed the right fuel at the correct times—and rest, so it could burn what it had already stored.

That accidental discovery became one of the most powerful tools in my weight loss journey. And now, I'm going to show you exactly how it works and how you can use it too.

The Science Behind Intermittent Fasting

So why does simply changing when you eat—not what you eat—make such a dramatic difference? The answer lies in how your body switches between two distinct metabolic states: fed and fasted.

The Metabolic Switch

Think of your body as having two fuel tanks: a small glucose tank (glycogen stored in your liver and muscles) and a massive fat tank (your body fat stores). When you eat frequently throughout the day, your body constantly runs on the glucose tank, and it never needs to tap into fat storage.

But when you fast for 12 to 16 hours, a metabolic shift occurs: your glucose tank empties, and your body flips a metabolic switch. It starts burning fat for fuel instead, producing molecules called ketones that provide clean, efficient energy for your brain and body.

This switch is where the magic happens. Insulin levels drop. Fat-burning hormones like growth hormone and norepinephrine increase. Your cells activate autophagy, a cellular cleanup process that removes damaged components and promotes longevity.

Without this fasting period, your body stays in constant fed-state mode—insulin remains elevated, fat-burning is suppressed, and your cells never get the deep rest and repair that comes from periodic fasting.

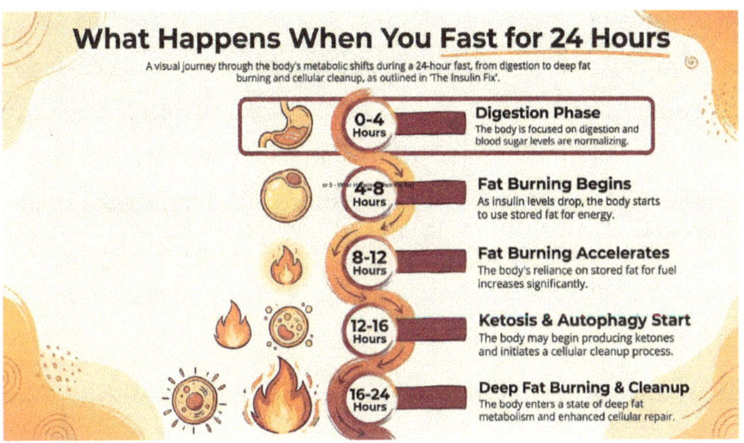

The Research That Proves It Works

Multiple studies have confirmed the power of intermittent fasting.

Study 1: Flipping the Metabolic Switch

Research published in the journal *Obesity* by Dr. Stephen Anton and colleagues examined how intermittent fasting triggers a metabolic shift from glucose to fat as an energy source. The study showed that after 12 to 16 hours of fasting, the body depletes glycogen stores and begins producing ketones from fat breakdown. This metabolic switch not only promotes weight loss but also improves insulin sensitivity, reduces inflammation, and enhances cellular stress resistance. The researchers concluded that intermittent fasting fundamentally changes how your body produces and uses energy.

Study 2: Health Benefits Beyond Weight Loss

A landmark review published in the *New England Journal of Medicine* by Dr. Rafael de Cabo and Dr. Mark Mattson examined decades of research on intermittent fasting. The findings were remarkable: intermittent fasting improved insulin sensitivity, reduced blood pressure, decreased oxidative stress, and enhanced cognitive function—even in people who didn't lose weight. The study demonstrated that the benefits of fasting extend far beyond calorie restriction, triggering powerful cellular and hormonal changes that promote health and longevity.

Study 3: Early Time-Restricted Feeding and Insulin Sensitivity

A controlled trial published in *Cell Metabolism* studied men with prediabetes who practiced early time-restricted feeding (eating within an eight-hour window ending in the afternoon). Even without weight loss, participants experienced dramatic improvements: insulin sensitivity increased, blood pressure dropped, and oxidative stress decreased. The researchers found that when you eat matters as much as what you eat, and that aligning eating with circadian rhythms amplifies metabolic benefits.

Study 4: Long-Term Effects on Body Composition

A comprehensive review in *Nutrition Reviews* analyzed multiple studies on intermittent fasting and body composition. The results showed that intermittent fasting preserves lean muscle mass while preferentially burning fat—unlike traditional calorie restriction, which often leads to muscle loss. Participants lost an average of three to eight percent of body weight over three to 24 weeks, with most of the weight loss coming from fat, not muscle. The review concluded that intermittent fasting is a sustainable, muscle-preserving approach to fat loss.

Study 5: Autophagy and Cellular Renewal

Research published in *Cell Metabolism* by Dr. Valter Longo and Dr. Mark Mattson explored how fasting activates autophagy—the cellular cleanup process that removes damaged proteins and organelles. The study showed that fasting for 16 to 24 hours triggers autophagy in multiple organs, including the brain, promoting cellular renewal and potentially reducing the risk of neurodegenerative diseases like Alzheimer's. The researchers described fasting as "putting your cells through a deep cleaning cycle" that may extend healthspan and lifespan.

The science is precise: intermittent fasting isn't just about eating less—it's about giving your body the metabolic rest it needs to burn fat, repair cells, and optimize health.

What Is Intermittent Fasting?

Intermittent fasting isn't a diet—it's an eating pattern. Instead of focusing on *what* you eat, it focuses on *when* you eat.

The concept is simple: you alternate between eating and fasting. During the fasting window, you consume no calories (or very minimal calories). During the eating window, you eat normally—focusing on nutrient-dense, low-glycemic foods.

It works because when you eat, your body releases insulin to process the glucose from your food. As we've discussed extensively, elevated insulin levels put your body in a fat-storage mode, preventing you from accessing stored fat for energy.

But when you fast—when you go an extended period without eating—your insulin levels drop. And when insulin drops, your body can finally unlock those fat stores and use them for fuel.

Think of it like this: every time you eat, you're making a "deposit" into your energy account. But if you're constantly eating (breakfast, snack, lunch, snack, dinner, snack), you're continually making deposits and never making withdrawals. Fasting gives your body time to make withdrawals—to burn the stored fat you've been carrying around.

Additionally, research suggests that extended fasting periods may trigger other beneficial processes:

- Improved insulin sensitivity. Your cells become more responsive to insulin. A study published in *Cell Metabolism* found that even without weight loss, early time-restricted feeding improved insulin sensitivity by up to 34 percent in men with prediabetes, demonstrating that fasting's metabolic benefits are independent of calorie restriction.
- Increased fat oxidation. Your body becomes more efficient at burning fat. Research published in *Obesity* demonstrates that after 12 to 16 hours of fasting, the body depletes glycogen

stores and shifts to burning fat for fuel, producing ketones that provide clean energy for the brain and body. This metabolic switch is key to sustainable fat loss.

- Increased autophagy, a cellular "cleaning" process that removes damaged cells and proteins. Studies published in *Cell Metabolism* and *Autophagy* show that fasting for 16 to 24 hours triggers autophagy across multiple organs, including the brain, promoting cellular renewal and potentially reducing the risk of neurodegenerative diseases such as Alzheimer's. Scientists describe this as "putting your cells through a deep cleaning cycle."

- Reduced inflammation. Chronic inflammation is linked to obesity and metabolic disease. A comprehensive review in the *New England Journal of Medicine* found that intermittent fasting significantly reduces inflammatory markers like C-reactive protein and IL-6, even in people who don't lose weight, suggesting that fasting has direct anti-inflammatory effects independent of fat loss.

- Increased mental clarity. Many people report enhanced focus and cognitive function while fasting. Research published in the *Annual Review of Nutrition* shows that ketones produced during fasting serve as superior fuel for the brain, improving cognitive performance, protecting neurons from damage, and enhancing mental clarity. Studies also show increased production of Brain-Derived Neurotrophic Factor (BDNF), a protein that supports brain health and neuroplasticity.

The Different Intermittent Fasting Protocols

There are several ways to practice intermittent fasting. Here are the most common, listed from easiest to most challenging:

12:12—The Beginner's Protocol

What it is: 12 hours fasting, 12 hours eating

Example: Finish dinner by 7 p.m.; don't eat again until 7 a.m.

Who it's for: Complete beginners, people transitioning from constant eating

My take: This is a great starting point. It's gentle enough that most people don't even notice they're "fasting"—you're essentially just eliminating late-night snacking and eating breakfast at a normal time (breaking the fast). But even this modest approach provides your body with 12 hours of metabolic rest, which can be beneficial.

14:10—The Next Step

What it is: 14 hours fasting, 10 hours eating

Example: Finish dinner by 7 p.m.; don't eat until 9 a.m.

Who it's for: People who've mastered 12:12 and want to progress

My take: This is where you start to see more noticeable benefits. By pushing breakfast back a couple of hours, you're giving your body more time to be in a fasted state. This was where I naturally settled during my first few weeks of planned intermittent fasting.

16:8—The Sweet Spot (Most Popular)

What it is: 16 hours fasting, eight hours eating

Example: Finish dinner by 8 p.m.; don't eat until 12 p.m. (noon).

Who it's for: People comfortable with fasting who want sustainable, long-term results

My take: This is the gold standard for most people. It's challenging enough to produce significant results but sustainable enough to maintain for months or years. Research suggests this may be the optimal window for fat loss while preserving muscle mass and energy levels. This became my default pattern for years.

18:6—Advanced Protocol

What it is: 18 hours fasting, six hours eating

Example: Finish dinner by 8 p.m.; don't eat until 2 p.m.

Who it's for: Experienced fasters, people breaking through plateaus

My take: This is more aggressive and not suitable for beginners. It's not something I'd do every day long-term—it's a tool I'd use strategically.

20:4—Very Advanced (Also Called "Warrior Diet")

What it is: 20 hours fasting, four hours eating

Example: Finish dinner by 8 p.m.; don't eat until 4 p.m.

Who it's for: Very experienced fasters, short-term use only

My take: This is intense. I experimented with this occasionally during plateau-breaking periods, but it requires significant adaptation and isn't sustainable long-term for most people. If you try this, do it sparingly and listen carefully to your body.

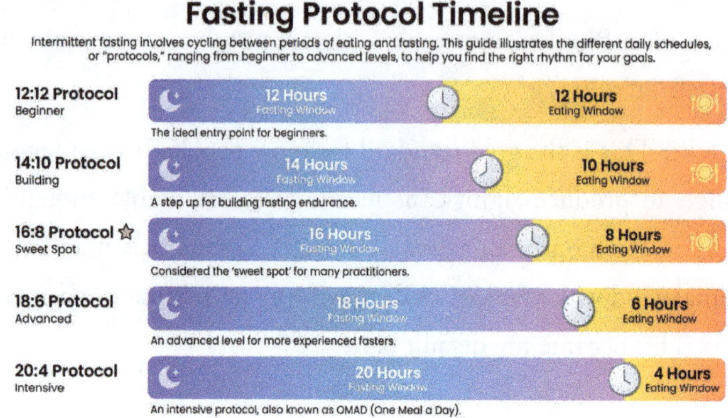

OMAD (One Meal A Day)

What it is: Eating all your calories in a single meal, then fasting for roughly 23 hours

Who it's for: Very experienced fasters with specific goals

My take: I never adopted this as a regular practice. While some people swear by it, I found it challenging to get adequate nutrition and variety in a single meal. If you try it, make that one meal as nutrient-dense as possible.

5:2—Alternate Day Approach

What it is: Eat normally five days per week, then restrict calories heavily (only eating 500 to 600 calories) on two non-consecutive days.

Who it's for: People who prefer periodic restriction rather than daily fasting

My take: I didn't use this approach personally, but I know people who've had great success with it. The advantage is that you're only "suffering" (if you want to call it that) for two days per week instead of a daily fasting window.

Which Protocol Should You Choose?

Here's my recommendation: Start with 12:12.

I can imagine that you are motivated and want to lose weight fast, but starting too aggressively is the fastest way to fail and give up entirely. Take your time.

The Progression:

Weeks 1 to 2: 12:12 (Eliminate late-night snacking and eat breakfast at a reasonable time)

Weeks 3 to 4: 14:10 (Push breakfast back 1 to 2 hours)

Weeks 5 to 8: 16:8 (The sweet spot—most people settle here)

Beyond Week 8: Experiment with 18:6 or 20:4 if needed for plateau-breaking, but only occasionally.

Master each level before progressing. If 14:10 feels difficult, stay there for a few more weeks before moving to 16:8. There's no reward for rushing, and you'll be more successful if you take your time.ee successful if you build gradually.

What You Can Have During Your Fasting Window

This is one of the most common questions about intermittent fasting: "What can I consume while fasting without breaking my fast?"

Here's your answer.

✅ **DOESN'T BREAK YOUR FAST:**

- Water. Drink plenty—this is essential. Eight to 10 glasses minimum.
- Black coffee. No milk, no cream, no sugar. Just black coffee. This became my morning ritual.
- Plain tea. Green tea, black tea, and herbal tea. Unsweetened, no milk.
- Sparkling water. As long as it's unsweetened and unflavored, or naturally flavored with no sweeteners.
- Electrolytes. If you're fasting for extended periods, adding salt, potassium, and magnesium to water can help prevent headaches and fatigue
- Apple cider vinegar, diluted in water (one tablespoon in eight ounces of water). This can actually help reduce hunger and may support blood sugar control.

❌ **BREAKS YOUR FAST:**

- Any solid food, obviously
- Milk or cream. Even a splash in your coffee triggers insulin.
- Any sweeteners. Sugar, honey, artificial sweeteners (even zero-calorie ones can trigger an insulin response in some people.

- Juice. This will give you a massive insulin spike—even "healthy" juices.
- Diet soda. Controversial, but the artificial sweeteners may trigger an insulin response in some people.
- Protein shakes. Definitely breaks your fast.
- Bone broth. Contains calories and protein—this breaks your fast (though some protocols allow it).
- Bulletproof coffee. This is coffee with butter and MCT oil. It's very popular in keto circles, but it absolutely breaks your fast because it contains calories and triggers fat metabolism.

My personal fasting toolkit:

- Black coffee in the morning (sometimes two or three cups).
- Water throughout the day (I'd aim for at least 10 glasses).
- Green tea in the afternoon if I needed variety.
- Occasionally, I would drink apple cider vinegar in water if I felt hungry.

When in doubt, stick to water, black coffee, or herbal tea. These are the safest bets. The goal during fasting is to keep insulin levels low and avoid triggering digestion.

How to Break Your Fast The Right Way

What you eat when you break your fast matters almost as much as the fasting itself. This is where many people sabotage their progress.

❌ The WRONG WAY to break a fast is with high-glycemic, processed foods, like:

- Sugary foods or drinks (juice, pastries, donuts, cereal)
- Large, heavy meals that overwhelm your digestive system
- Processed carbs (white bread, pasta, crackers)
- Fast food

After fasting, your insulin sensitivity is heightened. This is actually a good thing—it means your body is primed to use nutrients efficiently. But if you eat high-glycemic foods at this moment, you'll trigger an exaggerated blood sugar spike, followed by a crash, followed by intense cravings for more sugar. You'll undo much of the benefit of your fast.

✅ The Right Way to Break a Fast:

Break your fast gently, with nutrient-dense, low-glycemic foods—and follow the food order principle from Hack #1.

Why it's right: Even after a fast, the food order principle still applies; in fact, it's even *more* critical after fasting, because your digestive system has been resting and your insulin sensitivity is heightened.

By starting with vegetables, you:

- Protect your digestive tract with fiber
- Reduce the glucose spike from any foods that follow
- Maximize the metabolic benefits of your fast
- Stay in fat-burning mode longer

Give your body gentle, nutrient-dense fuel that keeps insulin stable and honors the natural sequence through which your body best processes food. You want to ease back into eating, not shock your system.

My Go-To Fast-Breaking Protocol:

12:00 p.m.: Small handful of raw spinach or a few cucumber slices
Give the digestive system a gentle wake-up call

12:05 p.m.: Eight to 10 raw almonds, eaten slowly
Add protein and healthy fat

12:15 p.m.: Large mixed-green salad with olive oil and lemon dressing
Main vegetable serving—establishes fiber mesh

12:25 p.m.: Grilled chicken thigh or salmon fillet
Primary protein and fat

12:35 p.m.: Small portion of roasted sweet potato (if still hungry—often, I skip this)
Optional carbs, only if genuinely needed

Seven Common Intermittent Fasting Mistakes (And How to Avoid Them)

Even with the best intentions, it's easy to stumble with intermittent fasting. Let's go over the seven mistakes I see most often (some of which I made myself!).

Mistake #1: Starting Too Aggressively

Jumping straight into 18:6, 20:4, or OMAD when you've never fasted before is a problem because your body needs time to adapt. Your hormones need to recalibrate. Your mental state needs to adjust. Going too hard too fast leads to misery, failure, and giving up entirely.

Start with 12:12. Seriously. Even if it feels "too easy," master it for at least a week. Then progress to 14:10 for another week or two. Then move to 16:8. Give yourself time to adapt at each level.

Remember, this is a marathon, not a sprint. Slow, steady progress wins.

Mistake #2: Not Drinking Enough Water

Forgetting to hydrate adequately during fasting windows causes dehydration. Dehydration amplifies hunger signals, causes headaches, leads to fatigue, and makes fasting feel miserable. Plus, many people mistake thirst for hunger.

Drink at least eight to 10 glasses of water during your fasting window—more if you're active, or it's hot outside. Keep a water bottle with you at all times. Add electrolytes (salt, potassium, magnesium) if you're fasting for extended periods (18+ hours) to prevent imbalances.

I'd drink two to three glasses of water first thing in the morning, another two to three mid-morning, and continue throughout the day. Sometimes I'd add a pinch of sea salt for electrolytes.

Mistake #3: Breaking Your Fast with Junk Food

Fasting all day, then eating pizza, ice cream, donuts, or other high-glycemic processed foods spikes your insulin dramatically. This triggers a blood sugar roller coaster—high spike, crash, intense cravings. You undo much of the benefit of your fast and set yourself up for overeating and poor choices the rest of the day.

Plan your first meal. Make it nutrient-dense, protein-rich, and aligned with Hacks #1 and #2. Break your fast gently with nuts or eggs, then eat a vegetable-first meal.

Remember, fasting gives you a metabolic advantage—don't waste it with poor food choices.

Mistake #4: Ignoring Hunger vs. Habit

Most of the time when you feel "hungry" during fasting, it's not actual hunger—it's habit ("it's breakfast time!"), boredom, stress, or social cues. If you respond to every "hunger" signal, not distinguishing between true physical hunger and habitual, emotional, or social eating triggers, you'll never build fasting endurance.

Learn to distinguish true hunger from habit.

TRUE HUNGER:

- Builds gradually over time
- Has physical sensations (stomach growling, slight fatigue)
- Will accept any food (even plain vegetables)
- Can wait 15 to 30 minutes without distress
- Happens three to five hours after the last meal

HABIT/EMOTIONAL EATING:

- Comes on suddenly
- Is a mental urge, not a physical sensation
- Brings on cravings for specific foods (usually carbs/sweets)
- Feels urgent, "must eat NOW."
- Happens at specific times regardless of the last meal

What to do:

- If true hunger, eat! Your body needs fuel.
- If habitual, drink water, wait 15 minutes, and distract yourself (walk, hobby, call a friend). Usually it passes.

Mistake #5: Being Rigidly Inflexible

Rigidly sticking to your fasting window no matter what—even when your body is genuinely struggling, you have exceptional circumstances, or it's causing problems in your life—breeds resentment and burnout. Life happens. Social events happen. Your body needs change day to day. If you treat fasting like an inflexible prison, you'll eventually rebel against it.

Be flexible. Permit yourself to adjust based on:

- How you feel (genuinely exhausted? Eat.)
- Social situations (family brunch? Enjoy it.)
- Special occasions (holidays, celebrations)
- Your menstrual cycle (women often need more flexibility)
- High-activity days (long hike? Fuel appropriately.)

Remember, you're building a lifestyle, not serving a sentence. Flexibility is what makes this sustainable in the long term.

Mistake #6: Fasting Every Single Day Without Breaks

Never varying your fasting pattern, doing the same window every single day for months on end, will result in your body getting too used to fasting. Your body is incredibly adaptive. If you do the same thing every day, your metabolism adjusts to that pattern. Weight loss can stall because your body has figured out the game.

Build in variety and breaks:

- Some days, fast longer (18:6)
- Some days, fast shorter (14:10)
- Some days, don't fast at all
- Consider cycling through intensive weeks and maintenance weeks
- Take occasional one- or two-week breaks from fasting entirely

It's a paradox: sometimes the best way to get results from fasting is to take a break from fasting. It keeps your body guessing and prevents metabolic adaptation.

Mistake #7: Using Fasting as an Excuse to Overeat

Intermittent fasting is not a license to binge. While you don't need to count calories, you still need to eat reasonable portions and choose quality foods. Thinking, "I fasted all day, so I can eat whatever I want now!" and then overcompensating by consuming enormous portions or junk food can negate the calorie deficit and blood sugar benefits of fasting.

The solution:

- Eat until you're satisfied (about 80 percent full), not stuffed
- Focus on nutrient-dense, whole foods
- Continue using food order (vegetables first)
- Continue choosing low-glycemic options
- Listen to your body's satiety signals

The truth: Fasting + smart eating = results. Fasting + junk food = disappointment.

Should You Exercise While Fasting?

This is one of the most common questions I get, and the answer is nuanced.

The short answer is that it depends on the type of exercise and on how well you are adapted to fasting.

Low-Intensity Exercise (Walking, Yoga, Stretching, Light Cardio)

- ☑ Generally fine during fasting
- ☑ May even enhance fat-burning (your body taps into fat stores for fuel)

I'd regularly take 30- to 60-minute walks during my fasting window. It felt great, suppressed appetite, and probably enhanced fat burning. No issues whatsoever.

Moderate-Intensity Exercise (Jogging, Cycling, Swimming)

⚠ Can work once you're fat-adapted (your body is efficient at using fat for fuel)

⚠ May feel harder at first if you're new to fasting

After a few months of fasting, moderate cardio during fasting periods felt fine. But in the early weeks, I sometimes felt light-headed or weak. I adjusted the timing or ate first.

High-Intensity Exercise (HIIT, Heavy Lifting, Sprinting, Competitive Sports)

⚠ Very challenging while fasting for most people

⚠ Hightened risk of feeling weak, dizzy, or unable to perform well

⚠ Consider timing workouts at the end of your eating window or right after breaking your fast

Once I was adapted to fasting (after about two or three months), I could do my seven-minute morning Tabata during my fasting window with no issues. Drinking black coffee before helped. With heavy weightlifting, I preferred to eat first, then train a few hours later.

The key principle: performance matters. If you're training for strength, power, or athletic performance, fueling appropriately before intense workouts is smart. If your primary goal is fat loss and you're doing lighter exercise, training during a fast can work well.

What About Post-Workout?

After intense exercise, break your fast with protein and carbs to support recovery (eggs, chicken, sweet potato).

After light exercise, follow standard fast-breaking protocol (vegetables first, small protein/fat serving, then carbs).

Special Considerations for Women

Women's hormonal cycles can significantly affect how they respond to intermittent fasting. This is important to understand and respect.

Female hormones (estrogen, progesterone) fluctuate throughout the menstrual cycle, and these fluctuations affect hunger, energy, metabolism, and how the body responds to stress (including the stress of fasting).

During certain phases of the menstrual cycle, particularly the luteal phase (the two weeks before your period), many women might experience:

- Increased hunger and cravings
- Lower energy levels
- Greater sensitivity to stress (including fasting stress)
- The body is preparing for a potential pregnancy (which makes it resistant to calorie restriction)

Fasting during the luteal phase can feel significantly harder than during the follicular phase (the two weeks after your period starts). Your body is literally fighting you because it's hormonally prioritizing different goals.

Recommendations for Women:

1. Start Even More Conservatively Than Men

Begin with 12:12 or at most 14:10, not 16:8. Give your body time to adapt without overwhelming your hormonal system.

2. Track Your Cycle

Pay attention to how fasting feels during different phases of your menstrual cycle:

- Follicular phase (days 1-14): You may find fasting easier, have more energy, and feel more mentally sharp
- Luteal phase (days 15-28): You may find fasting harder, feel hungrier, and have less energy

3. Be Flexible with Your Fasting Window

Adjust based on where you are in your cycle:

- Follicular phase: You might comfortably do 16:8 or even 18:6
- Luteal phase: You might need to shorten to 12:12 or 14:10, or take a break from fasting entirely

4. Consider "Crescendo Fasting."

Instead of fasting every day, fast for two or three non-consecutive days per week. This gives your body regular breaks and reduces hormonal stress. For example: fast Monday, Wednesday, and Friday. Eat normally on Tuesday, Thursday, Saturday, and Sunday.

5. Prioritize Nutrient Density

When you do eat, make it count. Focus on nutrient-dense foods that support hormonal health:

- Healthy fats (crucial for hormone production)
- Quality protein
- Iron-rich foods (women lose iron during menstruation)
- Magnesium and B vitamins (support hormone balance)

Red Flags to Watch For

If you experience any of these symptoms, stop fasting immediately and consult your healthcare provider:

- ❌ Irregular or missed periods (amenorrhea)
- ❌ Extreme fatigue that doesn't improve with rest
- ❌ Persistent hair loss
- ❌ Loss of libido
- ❌ Chronic insomnia
- ❌ Increased anxiety or depression
- ❌ Feeling cold all the time
- ❌ Significant mood swings

These can be signs that fasting is causing hormonal disruption. Your health is more important than any weight loss goal.

The Bottom Line for Women:

Intermittent fasting can work beautifully for women, but it requires more individualization, more flexibility, and more attention to hormonal signals than it typically does for men.

Honor your body's unique needs. What works for your male partner or friend might not work the same way for you, and that's normal.

Listening to Your Body: The Most Important Rule

I've given you a lot of information in this chapter—different protocols, timing strategies, tips, and tricks. But here's the single most crucial principle that overrides everything else:

Listen to your body.

Intermittent fasting should make you feel better, not worse. If you're consistently feeling:

- ✗ Extremely weak or dizzy
- ✗ Unable to focus or think clearly
- ✗ Irritable and angry (beyond customary initial adjustment)
- ✗ Anxious or depressed
- ✗ Obsessed with food
- ✗ Like you're developing an unhealthy relationship with eating

Then stop. Or adjust. Shorten your fasting window. Take breaks. Experiment with different timing.

There's no prize for suffering. The goal is sustainable, healthy weight loss and improved metabolic health—not punishment or deprivation.

Good signs that intermittent fasting is working for you:

- ✓ Increased mental clarity and focus
- ✓ Stable energy throughout the day
- ✓ Reduced cravings, especially for sugar
- ✓ Better mood and emotional stability

☑ Steady, sustainable weight loss
☑ Feeling empowered and in control around food
☑ Improved sleep quality
☑ Enhanced sense of well-being

If you're experiencing some or all of those benefits, that's your body telling you this approach is working. Keep going.

Quick-Win Challenge: Your First Week of Intermittent Fasting

Ready to try intermittent fasting? Here's your gentle introduction:

Days 1-3: The 12:12 Foundation

Eliminate eating after dinner and before breakfast: no late-night snacks, no early-morning eating.

Example:

- Finish dinner by 7:00 p.m.
- Don't eat again until 7:00 a.m.

What you can have during fasting: Water, black coffee, plain tea

What to notice: How does it feel? Are you genuinely hungry in the morning, or is it just a habit to eat when you wake?

Days 4-7: Stretch to 14:10

Push breakfast back by two hours.

Example:

- Finish dinner by 7:00 p.m.
- Don't eat again until 9:00 a.m.

During fasting: Water, black coffee, plain tea. Stay busy.

When you break your fast: Start with a small protein/fat serving (nuts, egg), then eat a vegetable-first meal.

What to track:

- Energy levels (1-10 scale)
- Hunger levels (1-10 scale)
- Mental clarity (1-10 scale)
- How quickly you adapted

End of Week Assessment:

Answer these questions:

1. How did I feel during fasting windows?
2. Was it easier or more complicated than I expected?
3. Did I notice any changes in hunger, energy, or mood?
4. Do I want to continue and progress to 16:8?

If the answer to Question 4 is YES, continue with 14:10 for another week, then try 16:8.

If the answer is NO or "I'm not sure," that's okay! Stay at 12:12 or 14:10 for as long as you need. Or take a break and revisit later. There's no rush.

Why This Hack Is So Powerful

Intermittent fasting is powerful because it:

- ☑ Gives your body metabolic rest. When insulin levels drop, fat-burning can increase.
- ☑ May simplify your life—fewer meals to plan, shop for, and cook.
- ☑ Can enhance mental clarity. Many people report better focus while fasting.
- ☑ Works synergistically with Hacks #1 and #2. Food order + low-glycemic swaps + fasting = metabolic optimization.
- ☑ May improve insulin sensitivity. Your cells become more responsive to insulin.
- ☑ Can accelerate fat loss. When combined with Hack #1 and Hack #2, the results can be dramatic.
- ☑ Supports cellular health. Research suggests autophagy and other repair processes may be activated.
- ☑ Builds discipline and body awareness. You learn to distinguish true hunger from habit.

When I reflect on losing 80 pounds and keeping it off, intermittent fasting was absolutely crucial. It was the strategy that broke through plateaus, eliminated cravings, and made weight maintenance almost effortless.

What's Next?

You now have a powerful tool to accelerate fat loss and improve metabolic health: intermittent fasting. But remember, it's just one tool in your toolbox. It works synergistically with food order (Hack #1) and low-glycemic swaps (Hack #2).

Start small. Be patient with yourself. Listen to your body. And adjust as needed.

Some people immediately thrive on intermittent fasting. Others take months to build up to it, and still others find that other approaches work better for their bodies. All of these outcomes are valid.

But here's what I can promise: if you combine intermittent fasting with wise food choices, something remarkable can happen. Your hunger may normalize. Your energy may stabilize. Your body may learn to access its fat stores efficiently, and weight loss can accelerate in a way that feels almost effortless.

Now, let's add the next layer: movement.

You don't need a gym membership or hours of cardio to lose weight and build a strong, healthy body. You need to turn your daily life into a fitness routine.

That's precisely what we'll explore in Chapter 6.

CHAPTER 6

HACK #4—TURN YOUR LIFE INTO A FITNESS ROUTINE

Here's a confession: I hate gyms.

The fluorescent lights. Waiting for the equipment. The monthly membership fees for a place I rarely wanted to go. The commute. The locker room awkwardness. The whole production of "going to work out."

And yet, for years, I believed that's what I had to do to lose weight and get fit. I thought exercise meant gym memberships, hour-long cardio sessions, and complicated workout routines.

I was wrong.

This is Hack #4: Turn Your Life Into a Fitness Routine—the strategy that helped me build sustainable movement into my daily life without ever setting foot in a gym.

You don't need expensive equipment. You don't need hours of free time. You don't need a gym membership or a personal trainer.

You need seven minutes in the morning, a basic understanding of how your body builds metabolic muscle, and a willingness to see everyday activities as opportunities for movement.

Let me show you how.

Important: Exercise Safety

Before starting any new exercise program, consult your healthcare provider, especially if you:

- Have any chronic health conditions
- Are over 50 and haven't been exercising regularly
- Have joint problems or injuries
- Take medications that affect heart rate or blood pressure

Start conservatively and build gradually. If you experience pain (not normal muscle fatigue), dizziness, or chest discomfort, stop immediately and consult a doctor.

Listen to your body, progress at your own pace, and prioritize safety over speed.

The Day I Discovered My Seven-Minute Solution

About eight months into my weight loss journey, I had a problem.

I was steadily losing weight using food order, low-glycemic swaps, and intermittent fasting. But I was also noticing something concerning: I was getting smaller, yet not getting stronger. My clothes fit better, but my body composition wasn't where I wanted it to be. I felt … soft.

I knew I needed to add exercise. But between four kids, a demanding career, and all the other demands of life, I genuinely didn't have time for hour-long gym sessions. Even 30 minutes felt like a luxury I couldn't afford most days.

So I started researching. What's the minimum effective dose of exercise for fat loss and muscle building?

That's when I discovered High-Intensity Interval Training (HIIT). And, more specifically, the Tabata protocol.

The concept seemed almost too good to be true: four minutes of intense exercise could potentially be more effective for fat loss than an hour of steady cardio. The research suggested that HIIT might trigger something called "EPOC"—Excess Post-Exercise Oxygen Consumption—also known as the "afterburn effect." Your body continues burning calories at an elevated rate for hours after the workout ends.

I was skeptical, but I was also desperate for something that would fit into my life.

So I tried it.

I used a free Tabata timer app for eight intervals: 20 seconds of work, 10 seconds of rest. I chose one bodyweight exercise (see list below) and stuck with it for all eight rounds. I'd go all-out for 20 seconds, rest for 10, then repeat—total time: four minutes.

The workout:

1. Jumping jacks
2. Squats
3. Push-ups (modified if needed)
4. High knees running in place
5. Lunges (alternating legs)
6. Mountain climbers
7. Burpees (modified if needed)
8. Plank hold

When the timer went off after four minutes, I was drenched in sweat, gasping for air, and feeling soreness in muscles I'd forgotten I had. I added a one-minute warm-up and a two-minute cool-down/stretch, bringing the total to seven minutes.

Seven minutes. That was it.

I committed to doing this every single morning for 30 days to see what would happen.

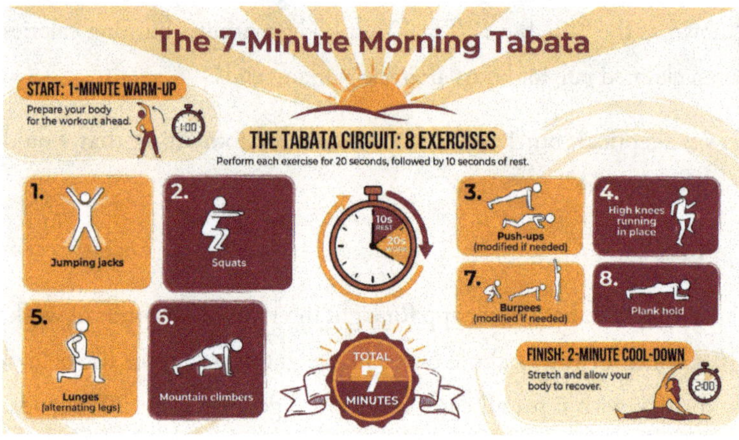

The Science Behind Movement and Metabolic Health

Why does something as simple as a ten-minute walk after meals make such a dramatic difference? The answer lies in how your muscles act like glucose sponges, soaking up blood sugar without requiring additional insulin.

The Muscle Glucose Uptake Effect

Think of your muscles as having two doors for glucose to enter: an insulin-dependent door and an insulin-independent door. When you're sitting still after a meal, only the insulin-dependent door is available—meaning your pancreas has to pump out lots of insulin to push glucose into cells.

But when you move—even gently—your biology works in your favor: your muscles open the insulin-independent door. They start pulling glucose directly from your bloodstream to fuel movement, bypassing the need for high insulin levels. It's like having an express lane that doesn't require the identical gatekeeper.

This muscle-driven glucose uptake happens within minutes of movement and continues for hours afterward. A simple 10- to 15-minute walk after eating can reduce your post-meal glucose spike by 30 to 50 percent, significantly lowering the insulin response.

Without this movement, all that post-meal glucose sits in your bloodstream, triggering a massive insulin surge that drives fat storage and sets you up for an energy crash later.

Multiple studies have confirmed the power of strategic movement:

Study 1: Post-Meal Walking Beats General Exercise

A randomized crossover study published in *Diabetologia* examined people with type 2 diabetes and compared post-meal walking to general daily activity. The results were striking: walking after meals was significantly more effective at lowering blood sugar than the same amount of walking spread throughout the day—just 10 minutes of walking after each main meal reduced 24-hour glucose levels and eliminated dangerous post-meal spikes. The researchers concluded that timing matters—post-meal movement is specifically powerful for glucose control.

Study 2: Exercise and Insulin Sensitivity

A comprehensive review published in the *International Journal of Sports Medicine* examined how exercise improves insulin sensitivity. The research showed that even a single bout of exercise makes cells more insulin-responsive for 24 to 48 hours afterward. Regular movement creates lasting improvements in how efficiently your body processes glucose, reducing the amount of insulin needed to maintain blood sugar control. The review demonstrated that exercise is one of the most potent non-pharmaceutical interventions for metabolic health.

Study 3: The Mind-Set Effect—Daily Activity Counts

A fascinating study published in *Psychological Science* examined hotel workers who performed physically demanding jobs but didn't consider themselves "exercisers." Researchers informed half the workers that their daily activities counted as excellent exercise. Four weeks later—without changing their behavior—the informed group showed significant improvements in blood pressure, body weight, and body composition. The study revealed that how we think about movement matters and that everyday activity has powerful health benefits when we recognize its value.

Study 4: High-Intensity Interval Training (HIIT)

Research published in the *Journal of Physiology* demonstrated that short bursts of high-intensity exercise—like the seven-minute Tabata protocol—produce remarkable metabolic adaptations. Studies showed that just four minutes of intense intervals improved insulin sensitivity, increased mitochondrial density (your cells' energy factories), and enhanced fat-burning capacity. The findings proved that you don't need hours of exercise—brief, intense movement triggers profound metabolic improvements.

Study 5: Exercise Guidelines for Diabetes Prevention

A joint position statement from the American College of Sports Medicine and the American Diabetes Association, published in *Diabetes Care*, reviewed decades of research on exercise and Type 2 diabetes. The conclusions were clear: both aerobic exercise (walking, cycling) and resistance training (strength exercises) independently improve glucose control and insulin sensitivity. The combination of both types of movement provides the most significant benefit. The guidelines emphasized that some movement is better than none, and that consistent daily activity is more important than intense occasional workouts.

The science is precise: movement is medicine for your metabolism, turning your muscles into powerful glucose-clearing tools that work independently of insulin.

What Happened After 30 Days of Seven-Minute Tabata

The results shocked me.

Week 1:

The first few days were brutal. I could barely make it to four minutes. My modified push-ups were embarrassing. My burpees looked more like flailing collapses than burpees. But I kept showing up.

Week 2:

I noticed I could do a few more reps in the 20-second windows. My form improved. I woke up sore but energized.

Week 3:

The workout started to feel ... almost easy? Not that it wasn't still hard—it was. But my body had adapted. I could push harder during the work intervals. My recovery improved.

Week 4:

I looked in the mirror and saw visible changes. My arms had definition. My legs looked more toned. My core was tighter. And I'd lost another four pounds that month—even though I was eating the same amount of food.

Seven minutes. Every morning. That's all it took.

But here's what made the most significant difference: consistency. Because it was only seven minutes, I never had an excuse to skip it. No matter how busy I was, I could find seven minutes before the kids woke up, before I showered, while my coffee brewed.

Seven minutes was doable. And doable meant sustainable.

My Seven-Minute Tabata Protocol: Step by Step

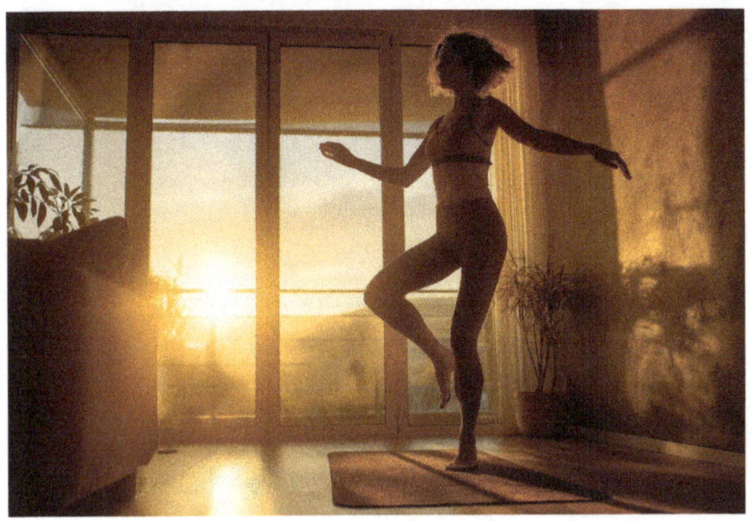

Here's the exact protocol I used (and still use today, over a decade later):

Equipment Needed:

- Timer (phone app works great—I use "Tabata Timer" apps)
- Small space (about 6x6 feet)
- Optional: yoga mat for comfort

The Warm-Up (one minute):

- 20 seconds: gentle jogging in place
- 20 seconds: arm circles (forward and back)
- 20 seconds: bodyweight squats (slow and controlled)

Purpose: Get your heart rate up gradually, warm your muscles, and prevent injury.

The Tabata (four minutes):

Structure: 20 seconds maximum effort → 10 seconds rest → repeat for eight rounds (four minutes total)

The Eight Exercises:

Round 1: Jumping Jacks

- 20 seconds: As many as you can, as fast as you can
- 10 seconds: Rest (stand still, breathe)

Round 2: Squats

- 20 seconds: Bodyweight squats, focus on form (feet shoulder-width, knees tracking over toes, chest up)
- 10 seconds: Rest

Round 3: Push-Ups

- 20 seconds: Standard push-ups (or modified on knees if needed—no shame, I started on my knees)
- 10 seconds: Rest

Round 4: High Knees

- 20 seconds: Run in place, bringing knees up toward chest as high and fast as possible
- 10 seconds: Rest

Round 5: Lunges

- 20 seconds: Alternating forward lunges (right leg, left leg, repeat)
- 10 seconds: Rest

Round 6: Mountain Climbers

- 20 seconds: Plank position, alternate driving knees toward chest rapidly
- 10 seconds: Rest

Round 7: Burpees

- 20 seconds: Squat down, hands on floor, jump feet back to plank, jump feet forward, stand up (jump at the top if you can)
- Modification: Step feet back/forward instead of jumping
- 10 seconds: Rest

Round 8: Plank Hold

- 20 seconds: Hold a strong plank position (forearms or hands, body straight)
- 10 seconds: Rest

The Cool-Down (two minutes):

Thirty seconds each:

- Standing forward fold (touch toes, stretch hamstrings)
- Quad stretch (standing, pull one foot to the butt, then switch)
- Chest/shoulder stretch (clasp hands behind back, lift arms)
- Child's pose or cat-cow stretch (if you're on the floor)

Purpose: Bring your heart rate down gradually, stretch warm muscles, and prevent stiffness.

Total time: seven minutes.

That's it. Seven minutes every morning changed my body and my life.

Progression and Modifications

If you're a complete beginner, start with just two rounds (one minute of work) instead of all eight. Do this for a week. Then add two more rounds the following week. Build up gradually.

If 20 seconds feels too long, start with 15 seconds of work and 15 seconds of rest. It builds up over time.

If specific exercises are too complex:

- Push-ups: Do them on your knees, or against a wall
- Burpees: Step back instead of jumping, skip the jump at the end
- Mountain climbers: Go slower, focus on form
- Plank: Hold on your knees instead of toes

As you get stronger:

- Increase the intensity: jump higher, move faster, go deeper in squats
- Add light dumbbells to some exercises (squat with weights, lunges with weights)
- Extend to six or eight minutes (12 or 16 rounds)
- Do it twice per day (morning and evening) on days when you have extra energy

Something is always better than nothing. Even if you can only do two minutes at first, do two minutes. Consistency matters more than intensity when you're starting.

The Muscle Factor: Why Strength Training Matters More Than Cardio

About a year into my weight loss journey, I made another important discovery: building muscle was the key to long-term metabolic health.

Muscle tissue generally burns more calories at rest than fat tissue. A lot more:

- One pound of muscle burns about six to 10 calories per day at rest.
- One pound of fat burns about two to three calories per day at rest.

This might not sound like much, but it adds up. If you build 10 pounds of muscle, you're burning an additional 60 to 100 calories per day doing absolutely nothing. That's 420 to 700 calories per week. That's 1,800 to 3,000 calories per month. That's the equivalent of running 20 to 30 miles per month.

Muscle is your metabolic engine. The more you have, the more calories you burn 24/7, even while you sleep.

This is why people who build muscle find it easier to maintain their weight loss in the long term. Their metabolism is constantly working for them.

My Strength Training Journey

After about 10 months of Tabata and bodyweight exercises, I realized I needed to add resistance training to build significant muscle.

I still didn't want a gym membership, so I bought two things:

1.   A suspension trainer (straps that anchor to a door or beam—simple, versatile, highly effective)
2.   A pull-up bar that fits in a doorframe

Total cost: About $150-$200. One-time expense. No monthly fees.

I added two 20-minute strength sessions per week

STRENGTH SESSION A (TUESDAY): UPPER BODY

1. Suspension Push-Ups: three sets of as many reps as possible (AMRAP)
Feet in straps, hands on ground—or reverse for even more challenge

2. Suspension Rows: three sets of 10 to 12 reps
The classic suspension exercise—lean back and pull yourself up

3. Suspension Chest Press: three sets of 8 to 10 reps
Lean forward, arms extended, and lower yourself into a press

4. Suspension Bicep Curls: three sets of 10 to 12 reps
Lean back, palms up, curl your body toward your hands

5. Suspension Tricep Extensions: three sets of eight to 10 reps
Lean forward, elbows high, extend arms

6. Pull-Ups or Assisted Pull-Ups (using pull-up bar): three sets of as many reps as possible

Rest: 30 to 60 seconds between sets

Total time: 20 to 25 minutes

STRENGTH SESSION B (FRIDAY): LOWER BODY AND CORE

1. Suspension Squats: three sets of 10 to 12 reps
Hold straps for balance, squat deep

2. Suspension Single-Leg Deadlifts: three sets of 8 to 10 reps per leg
Hold straps, balance on one leg, hinge at the hips

3. Suspension Lunges: three sets of 10 reps per leg
Back foot elevated in a strap—intense quad and glute work

4. Calf Raises (bodyweight or holding something for balance): three sets of 15 to 20 reps

5. Suspension Plank (feet in straps): three sets of 30 to 60 seconds
Unstable surface = core on fire

6. Suspension Pike or Knee Tucks: three sets of 10 to 12 reps
Feet in straps, pull knees to chest or pike hips up

Rest: 30 to 60 seconds between sets

Total time: 20 to 25 minutes

Why This Worked for Me

- Minimal equipment. Two pieces of gear, one-time cost, no gym needed.
- Full-body engagement. The instability of suspension training means your core is working constantly, even during "arm" or "leg" exercises.

- Adjustable difficulty. As I got stronger, I just changed my body angle to make the exercises harder. No need to buy heavier weights.

- Portable. I could take the suspension trainer anywhere—on vacation, to the park, to a friend's house. My workout went wherever I went.

- Time-efficient. Two 20-minute sessions per week were enough to build and maintain muscle while supporting my weight loss.

The Results: What Strength Training Did for My Body

Within three months of adding suspension training, I underwent performance, metabolic, physical, and mindset changes.

Performance changes:

- My Tabata workouts felt easier because I was stronger
- Everyday tasks (carrying groceries, moving furniture, playing with kids) became effortless
- Energy levels stayed high throughout the day

Metabolic changes:

- Weight maintenance became easier—I could eat more without gaining
- My body composition improved dramatically (more muscle, less fat)
- I felt like my metabolism had been "awakened"

Physical changes:

- My arms looked more defined
- My chest and back developed visible muscle
- My core was noticeably stronger (hello, visible abs!)
- My posture improved dramatically

The mindset shift:

I stopped thinking about exercise as "burning calories" and started thinking about it as "building my metabolic engine." This reframe was huge. I wasn't punishing my body—I was strengthening it.

I wasn't trying to become a bodybuilder. I just wanted to look good, feel strong, and preserve muscle while losing fat.

Suspension training delivered precisely that.

Turn Your Daily Life Into a Fitness Routine

Formal exercise is just one small piece of the movement puzzle. The real magic happens when you start seeing your entire day as an opportunity to move.

I call this "lifestyle exercise," and it's how I stay active without ever feeling like I'm "working out."

Strategy 1: The Parking Lot Rule

Old habit: Driving around looking for the closest parking spot
New habit: Parking at the far end of the lot and walking

Why it matters:

- An extra two to five minutes of walking per trip
- If you run errands three or four times per week, that's six to twenty minutes of bonus walking
- Over a year: 300 to 1,000 extra minutes of movement
- Plus, you avoid parking lot stress and door dings

Strategy 2: The Stair Rule

Old habit: Taking elevators and escalators automatically

New habit: Always take the stairs

Why it matters:

- Stair-climbing is one of the most effective exercises for leg strength and cardiovascular health
- Burns significantly more calories than walking on flat ground
- Builds muscle in glutes, quads, and calves

My rule: If it's fewer than six floors, stairs are mandatory. No excuses.

Strategy 3: Turn Housework Into Exercise

This one changed everything for me. I stopped seeing chores as annoying tasks and began seeing them as opportunities for movement.

Vacuuming:

- Do lunges while you vacuum
- Engage your core and make it deliberate
- Thirty minutes of active vacuuming can burn 100 to 150 calories

Yard work:

- Raking leaves: squats and twisting movements
- Mowing the lawn: walking and pushing resistance
- Gardening: squatting, reaching, lifting

Washing dishes:

- Stand on one leg to work balance and core
- Do calf raises while scrubbing
- Engage your abs consciously

Laundry:

- Every time you move clothes from the washer to the dryer, do 10 squats
- Folding clothes: sit on the floor instead of a chair (requires more core engagement and makes getting up an exercise)

The mindset: Every movement counts. Stop thinking "I need to exercise." Start thinking, "I'm always exercising."

Strategy 4: Walking Meetings and Phone Calls

Whenever I had a phone call that didn't require me to be at my computer, I'd walk.

30-minute call = 30 minutes of walking = 100 to 150 calories burned + mental clarity boost

Over a week, multiple calls could add up to two to three hours of bonus walking without ever "going for a walk."

Strategy 5: Play With Your Kids (Or Pets)

Some of my best workouts came from simply playing actively with my children:

- Tag in the backyard
- Throwing a football or Frisbee
- Bike rides together
- Swimming
- Dancing in the living room
- Roughhousing (carefully!)

This wasn't "exercise." This was joy. But it burned hundreds of calories, built strength, and created memories.

If you have pets, the same principle: active play with your dog (fetch, running, wrestling) is excellent exercise that doesn't feel like work.

Strategy 6: The "Commercial Break" Challenge

When I watched TV, I'd use commercial breaks for movement:

- Push-ups
- Squats
- Plank holds
- Stretching

Two hours of TV with four to five commercial breaks = 10 to 15 minutes of exercise sprinkled throughout. Better than sitting motionless for two hours.

Strategy 7: Walk After Meals

Remember Hack #1 (food order)? Here's a bonus strategy that amplifies its benefits:

Walk for 10 to 15 minutes after dinner.

Research suggests that walking after meals can help lower post-meal blood sugar spikes. Muscle activity helps your body use glucose more efficiently, requiring less insulin.

This became a family ritual: after dinner, we'd all go for a short walk around the neighborhood. The kids loved it (energy release before bed), my wife and I got time to talk, and it supported my metabolic health.

Win-win-win.

The "I Don't Have Time" Excuse: Demolished

Let's do the math on my exercise routine:

Tabata (five days/week): 7 minutes x 5 = 35 minutes
Strength training (two days/week): 20 minutes x 2 = 40 minutes
Total formal exercise per week: 75 minutes (1 hour and 15 minutes)

Now add in lifestyle movement:

Parking far away: 10 minutes/week
Taking stairs: 10 minutes/week
Active housework: 20 minutes/week
Playing with kids: 60 minutes/week
Walking after dinner: 70 minutes/week (10 min x 7 days)
Total movement per week: 245 minutes (about four hours)

But most of that "lifestyle movement" wasn't extra time—it was time I was already spending. I was going to park somewhere, climb stairs (or take an elevator), do housework, and spend time with my kids anyway. I just made those activities more intentional and active.

The only "extra" time I carved out was 75 minutes per week for Tabata and strength training.

75 minutes per week. Ten to 11 minutes per day.

If you can't find 10 minutes per day, the problem isn't time—it's priorities.

The Importance of Rest and Recovery

Here's something I learned the hard way: more is not always better.

About 14 months into my journey, I got overly enthusiastic. I was seeing great results, so I thought, "If five days of Tabata is good, seven days must be better! And maybe I should do it twice a day!"

Bad idea.

Within two weeks, I was:

- Constantly exhausted
- Irritable and moody
- Not sleeping well
- Experiencing joint pain
- Actually gaining a little weight (my body was stressed and holding onto water/fat)

I was overtraining. My body wasn't getting enough time to recover and rebuild.

That's when I learned one of the most important lessons about exercise: Your body transforms during rest, not during the workout.

Why Rest Matters

When you exercise—especially intense exercise like Tabata or strength training—you're actually breaking down muscle tissue. Microscopic tears occur in the muscle fibers. This is normal and necessary—the magic happens afterward, during rest:

- Your body repairs the damaged muscle fibers
- It rebuilds them slightly stronger and larger than before (adaptation)
- Your central nervous system recovers
- Glycogen stores replenish
- Hormones rebalance

Without adequate rest, this process can't happen effectively. You keep breaking down without rebuilding. That's a recipe for injury, burnout, and stalled progress.

My Rest Guidelines:

1. At least one or two full rest days per week

These are days with no formal exercise—just normal daily movement (walking, housework, etc.). My body needs this time to recover.

2. Sleep seven to nine hours per night

This is non-negotiable. Sleep is when your body does most of its repair work. It's also when growth hormone is released—critical for muscle building and fat loss.

Poor sleep undermines everything else you're doing. Prioritize it.

3. Don't exercise when sick or exhausted

If you're fighting an illness or you're genuinely depleted, your body needs rest more than it needs exercise. Skip the workout. Recover. You'll come back stronger.

4. Listen to soreness

Normal muscle soreness (Delayed Onset Muscle Soreness, or DOMS) 24 to 48 hours after a workout is delicate. That's your muscles adapting.

But sharp pain, joint pain, or soreness that doesn't resolve after two or three days is a warning sign. Rest, ice, and if it persists, see a doctor.

5. Deload weeks

Every eight to 12 weeks, I take a "deload week" in which I reduce exercise intensity by about 50 percent. Maybe I do Tabata at 70 percent effort instead of 100 percent. Maybe I skip strength training entirely. This gives my body a chance to recover fully and prevents burnout.

Recovery Supports:

Beyond rest days and sleep, these strategies support recovery:

- Adequate protein intake. Your muscles need protein to repair. Aim for 0.8 to 1.2g per kilogram of body weight daily.

- Hydration. Water is essential for every recovery process in your body. Drink plenty.

- Stress management. Chronic stress (work, relationships, life) increases cortisol, which can interfere with recovery and fat loss. Find ways to manage stress, such as meditation, deep breathing, hobbies, and time in nature.

- Stretching and mobility work. Spend five to 10 minutes daily on gentle stretching or yoga. It improves flexibility, reduces injury risk, and helps with recovery.

The Bottom Line on Rest:

Exercise breaks down. Rest builds up. Both are essential.

If you're training hard but not seeing results, the problem might not be that you're not doing enough—it might be that you're not *resting* enough.

What About Traditional Cardio?

You might be wondering: "What about running? Cycling? Swimming? Traditional cardio?"

Honestly, I don't do much traditional steady-state cardio, and I don't think it's necessary for fat loss.

Here's why:

1. It's time-intensive.

To burn significant calories, you need at least 30 to 60 minutes. I don't have that time, and most people don't either.

2. It can increase appetite.

Traditional steady-state cardio can actually increase appetite for many people. Research published in Obesity found that moderate-intensity aerobic exercise often triggers compensatory eating, with participants consuming more calories after exercise than they burned during the workout. In contrast, high-intensity exercise and strength training tend to temporarily suppress appetite, making them more effective for weight loss.

3. It can lead to muscle loss.

Extended steady-state cardio, especially without adequate protein and strength training, can cause your body to break down muscle tissue for energy. This lowers your metabolic rate long-term.

4. There are diminishing returns.

Your body adapts quickly to steady-state cardio. After a few weeks, you burn fewer calories doing the same activity because your body becomes more efficient.

5. It doesn't build muscle.

Cardio maintains cardiovascular health, which is valuable, but it doesn't build the metabolic muscle that keeps you lean in the long term.

When Cardio Makes Sense:

I'm not anti-cardio. I'm just pro-efficiency.

Cardio is great if:

- You genuinely enjoy it (running, cycling, swimming for pleasure)
- You're training for a specific event (marathon, triathlon)
- You use it for stress relief and mental health (many people find running meditative)
- You're doing it socially (group classes, sports teams, biking with friends)

But if your only goal is fat loss and you don't particularly enjoy cardio?

Skip it. Focus on HIIT (like Tabata) and strength training instead. You'll get better results in less time.

Exercise Myths I Had to Unlearn

As I delved deeper into fitness, I realized how much misinformation is out there. Here are the myths I had to unlearn:

Myth #1: "You have to exercise for 30 to 60 minutes to see results."

Intensity matters more than duration. Seven minutes of high-intensity Tabata can potentially deliver fat-loss results similar to or better than 30 minutes of steady jogging.

Myth #2: "Cardio is the best exercise for weight loss."

Strength training builds muscle, which increases your resting metabolic rate. Long-term, muscle is more valuable for fat loss than cardio.

Myth #3: "You need a gym to get fit."

Bodyweight exercises are sufficient for most people. I built my best physique at home with minimal equipment.

Myth #4: "More exercise equals more results."

Rest and recovery are when your body actually transforms—overtraining leads to burnout, injury, and stalled progress.

Myth #5: "Exercise is the most important factor for weight loss."

Diet is far more important than exercise for weight loss. You can't out-exercise a bad diet. Exercise is powerful for body composition, health, and maintenance—but weight loss happens primarily in the kitchen.

Myth #6: "You should exercise every day."

Your body needs rest. Five or six days of exercise per week, with one or two full rest days, is generally optimal for most people.

Myth #7: "If you're not sore, you didn't work hard enough."

Soreness is not a reliable indicator of a good workout. As you adapt, you'll get less sore. That's normal and doesn't mean your workouts are less effective.

Quick-Win Challenge: Your First Week of Movement

Ready to start building your fitness routine? Here's your challenge for the next seven days:

Days 1 to 3: Master the Basics

Morning: Try the seven-minute Tabata protocol

- Start with just two to four rounds (one to two minutes) if needed
- Focus on learning the movements, not achieving perfection
- Modify exercises as necessary

Daily: Implement one lifestyle strategy

- Park far away from store entrances
- Take stairs instead of the elevator
- Do squats while brushing teeth

Track: How do you feel? Energy levels? Soreness? Enjoyment?

Days 4 to 7: Build Momentum

Morning: Increase to four to six rounds of Tabata (two to three minutes)

Daily: Add a second lifestyle strategy

- Walk 10 minutes after dinner
- Do bodyweight exercises during TV commercial breaks
- Turn housework into active movement

Optional: Try one 15 to 20-minute strength session if you have a suspension trainer or resistance bands for the beginning

End of Week Assessment:

Answer these questions:

1. What felt good about adding movement?
2. What felt challenging?
3. Which strategies fit most naturally into my life?
4. What will I continue next week?

Remember: You're not trying to transform overnight. You're building sustainable habits that will serve you for life.

Why This Hack Is So Powerful

Movement—when done intelligently and consistently—can be powerful because it:

- ✅ Builds metabolic muscle and increases your resting calorie burn 24/7.
- ✅ Preserves muscle during weight loss and ensures you're losing fat, not muscle.
- ✅ Improves insulin sensitivity by helping your body use glucose more efficiently.
- ✅ Enhances mood and energy. Exercise releases endorphins and reduces stress.
- ✅ Supports long-term maintenance by making it easier to keep weight off permanently.
- ✅ Fits into any lifestyle—no gym or huge time commitment required.
- ✅ Compounds over time—small daily actions create massive, long-term results.

As I consider my journey from 280 to 200 pounds, exercise wasn't the primary driver—diet and intermittent fasting were. But exercise was the strategy that transformed my body composition, gave me energy, and made maintenance effortless.

Most importantly, it didn't feel like a burden. It felt like a gift I gave myself every morning.

What's Next?

You now have the movement piece of the puzzle: your seven-minute Tabata protocol, strength training fundamentals, and strategies for turning daily life into fitness opportunities.

In the next chapter, everything we've learned so far comes together most powerfully.

CHAPTER 7

HACK #5—HEALTHY FATS AND THE KETOSIS SECRET

For decades, we've been told that fat makes you fat. Eating fat will clog your arteries, cause heart disease, and ruin your health. We've been told to eat low-fat everything—low-fat yogurt, low-fat salad dressing, fat-free cookies.

It was all wrong.

Fat isn't the enemy. In fact, for me, fat became the secret weapon that eliminated my cravings, stabilized my energy, and turned my body into a fat-burning machine.

This is Hack #5: Healthy Fats and The Ketosis Secret.

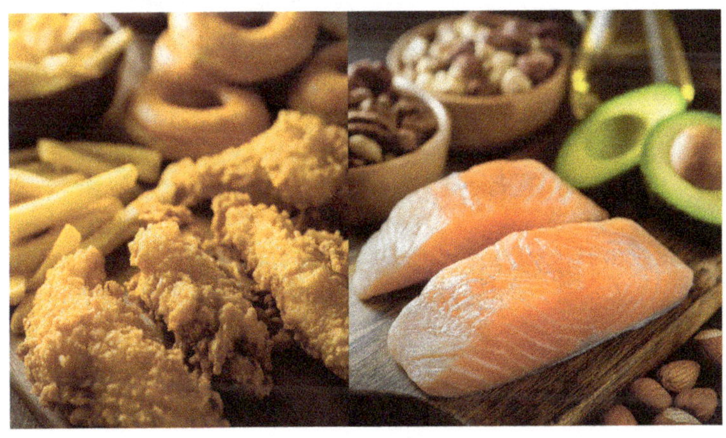

In this chapter, you'll discover why healthy fats are essential for weight loss, how to choose the right fats, and how a metabolic state called ketosis can potentially eliminate hunger and cravings in a way nothing else can.

This was the hack that changed everything for me. Let me show you why.

Important: Ketogenic Diets and Medical Conditions

If you have any of the following conditions, consult your healthcare provider before significantly increasing fat intake or attempting ketosis:

- Diabetes (Type 1 or Type 2) or Pre-Diabetes
- Liver disease
- Pancreatic conditions
- Gallbladder issues or history of gallstones
- Heart disease or high cholesterol

Also, consult your healthcare provider if you take any other medications for chronic conditions.

Ketosis is not appropriate for everyone. This chapter provides information about the author's experience, and it is not medical advice.

The Science Behind Healthy Fats and Ketosis

So why does eating more fat help you burn fat? It sounds counterintuitive, but the answer lies in how fat fundamentally changes your metabolism and switches your body from a sugar-burner to a fat-burner.

The Fat-Adaptation Effect

Think of your body as a hybrid car with two fuel systems: one that runs on glucose (sugar) and one that runs on fat (ketones). For most people eating the standard high-carb diet, the glucose engine runs constantly while the fat engine sits idle—even though you're carrying gallons of fuel (body fat) that never gets used.

When you reduce carbohydrates and increase healthy fats, your body adapts to burn fat preferentially for fuel. Your liver starts converting fatty acids into ketones—clean-burning molecules that your brain and body can use for energy. This metabolic state is called ketosis.

In ketosis, insulin levels drop dramatically. Your cells become exquisitely sensitive to insulin again. Fat cells release stored energy instead of hoarding it. Hunger decreases because fat and ketones provide steady, long-lasting fuel—unlike the blood sugar roller coaster of carb-heavy eating.

Without adequate healthy fats, your body stays dependent on glucose, requiring frequent meals to maintain energy. Insulin remains elevated, fat-burning is suppressed, and you're trapped in a cycle of hunger and cravings.

The Research That Proves It Works

Study 1: Low-Carb Beats Low-Fat for Weight Loss

A landmark randomized controlled trial published in the *Annals of Internal Medicine* compared a low-carbohydrate, ketogenic diet to a traditional low-fat diet for treating obesity and high cholesterol. After six months, the low-carb group lost significantly more weight, had greater reductions in triglycerides, and showed larger increases in HDL (good cholesterol), despite eating more total fat and saturated fat. The study challenged decades of conventional wisdom, demonstrating that dietary fat doesn't make you fat when insulin is controlled.

Study 2: Beyond Weight Loss—Therapeutic Benefits of Ketogenic Diets

A comprehensive review published in the *European Journal of Clinical Nutrition* examined the therapeutic uses of very-low-carbohydrate (ketogenic) diets beyond weight loss. The research documented improvements in epilepsy, Type 2 diabetes, polycystic ovary syndrome (PCOS), acne, and even some cancers. The review showed that ketogenic diets reduce inflammation, improve mitochondrial function, and stabilize brain chemistry. The authors concluded that ketosis offers profound metabolic and neurological benefits that extend far beyond fat loss.

Study 3: Ketones as Brain Fuel

Research published in the *Annual Review of Nutrition* by Drs. John Newman and Eric Verdin explored how beta-hydroxybutyrate (the primary ketone body) functions as a signaling molecule. The study showed that ketones don't just fuel the brain—they also reduce inflammation, protect neurons from damage, enhance mitochondrial efficiency, and may improve cognitive function. Many people report dramatic mental clarity and focus in ketosis. The researchers described ketones as "a superior fuel for the brain" compared to glucose.

Study 4: Low-Carb Reduces Inflammation Better Than Low-Fat

A study published in the journal *Lipids* compared low-fat and low-carbohydrate diets with respect to markers of inflammation and cardiovascular health. Despite higher saturated fat intake, the low-carb group showed significantly greater reductions in inflammatory markers and improvements in triglycerides and HDL cholesterol. The research demonstrated that when carbohydrate intake and insulin levels are controlled, dietary fat—even saturated fat—doesn't drive inflammation or heart disease risk.

Study 5: Saturated Fat and Heart Disease—Reassessing the Evidence

A groundbreaking meta-analysis published in the *American Journal of Clinical Nutrition* examined 21 prospective studies involving nearly 350,000 participants. The shocking conclusion: there was no significant association between saturated fat intake and heart disease, stroke, or cardiovascular mortality. This landmark study challenged 50 years of dietary dogma and suggested that the war on saturated fat may have been misguided—especially when saturated fat is consumed in the context of low-carbohydrate, insulin-controlled eating.

Study 6: The Art and Science of Low-Carb Living

In their comprehensive book, Drs. Jeff Volek and Stephen Phinney compiled decades of research on ketogenic diets and fat metabolism. Their work demonstrated that well-formulated low-carb, high-fat diets preserve lean muscle mass, enhance athletic performance, improve metabolic markers, and promote sustainable fat loss. They showed that fat-adaptation takes two to four weeks, but results in profound metabolic advantages: stable energy, reduced hunger, mental clarity, and efficient fat-burning. Their research proved that eating fat doesn't make you fat—eating fat in the presence of high insulin does. The science is precise: healthy fats aren't the enemy—they're the solution to breaking free from insulin-driven fat storage and reclaiming metabolic flexibility.

The Truth About Cravings: They Can Change

Before I dive into ketosis and healthy fats, I need you to understand something fundamental: Any craving can be changed.

I know that sounds impossible. Maybe right now you're thinking, "I've always craved chocolate. I've always needed bread. I can't imagine life without ice cream."

I felt the same way.

For most of my life, I was controlled by cravings. I craved sugar constantly. Chocolate called to me every afternoon. Ice cream was my nightly ritual. Bread was non-negotiable. These weren't just passing desires—they felt like deep, biological needs that defined who I was.

I assumed these cravings were permanent. Part of my personality. Just "how I was wired."

But I was utterly wrong.

Your Body Adapts to Whatever You Feed It

Cravings aren't permanent traits. They're adaptations.

Your body learns to crave whatever fuel you regularly give it:

- If you feed it sugar consistently, it craves sugar.
- If you feed it processed carbs consistently, it craves processed carbs.
- If you feed it healthy fats consistently, it learns to crave healthy fats.

Your taste buds, your gut bacteria, your hormonal signals, your brain's reward pathways—they all adapt based on what you eat most often.

The problem? Most of us have been feeding our bodies sugar and refined carbs for decades. So naturally, that's what we crave. Our bodies are simply asking for more of what we've trained them to expect.

The solution? Retrain your body with different fuels.

The Adaptation Timeline: What to Expect

Here's what research and my own experience taught me about changing cravings:

Weeks 1 to 2: The Hardest Phase

This is when you're fighting against years—maybe decades—of established patterns. Your taste buds expect certain flavors. Your brain expects certain rewards. You'll feel resistance, perhaps even mild withdrawal symptoms.

This is normal. This is temporary. And you can get through it.

Weeks 3 to 4: The Shift Begins

Foods that once seemed bland start tasting good. The intense cravings begin to fade. You notice you can go longer without thinking about food.

Weeks 5 to 8: The Recalibration

Your body has adapted. Foods you once found irresistible now seem too sweet, too heavy, even unappealing. Foods that once seemed dull now taste delicious. Your cravings have shifted from working against you to working for you.

Research suggests it takes an average of 66 days to form a new habit—though it can range from 18 to 254 days depending on the person and the complexity of the behavior.

The key insight: You don't have to white-knuckle through cravings forever. You need to push through the initial two to four weeks while your body adapts.

Why This Matters for You

If you're struggling with cravings right now, I want you to know:

Those cravings are not permanent.
They are not who you are.
They will change.
You're not weak. You're not broken. You're not lacking willpower.
Your body is simply asking for the fuel it's been trained to expect.

When you change the fuel—when you embrace healthy fats and potentially enter ketosis—your cravings will change too.

And that's when weight loss stops being a battle and starts becoming effortless.

This realization became the foundation of my approach to healthy fats and ketosis.

Let me show you exactly how it works.

What Is Ketosis?

Ketosis is a metabolic state in which your body primarily burns fat for fuel rather than carbohydrates.

Under normal circumstances—when you eat a standard diet with regular carbohydrate intake—your body's preferred fuel source is glucose (sugar). Every time you eat carbs, they're broken down into glucose, which enters your bloodstream. Your pancreas releases insulin to shuttle that glucose into your cells for energy.

But when you significantly reduce carbohydrate intake (typically to under 50 grams per day, sometimes lower), your body runs out of readily available glucose. Since it still needs energy to function, it does what humans have done for millions of years during times of food scarcity: it starts breaking down stored fat into molecules called ketones.

Ketones become an alternative fuel source for your brain, muscles, and organs. Your body shifts from being a "sugar-burner" to a "fat-burner."

This is nutritional ketosis.

Nutritional Ketosis vs. Ketoacidosis

Let me be very clear: Nutritional ketosis is NOT the same as diabetic ketoacidosis.

Nutritional Ketosis:

- A natural metabolic state
- Ketone levels: 0.5-3.0 mmol/L
- Safe and beneficial for most people
- How humans survived periods without food throughout evolution

Diabetic Ketoacidosis (DKA):

- A dangerous medical emergency
- Ketone levels: >10 mmol/L (often much higher)
- Occurs primarily in people with Type 1 diabetes when insulin is absent
- Requires immediate medical treatment

If you have Type 1 diabetes, you should NOT attempt ketosis without close medical supervision. For everyone else, nutritional ketosis is generally safe—but always consult your doctor if you have any health conditions.

Nutritional Ketosis vs. „Keto Diet"

There's also a difference between the metabolic state of ketosis and the rigid "keto diet" popularized online.

Nutritional Ketosis (what this chapter discusses):

- A metabolic state where your body efficiently burns fat for fuel
- Can be achieved through various approaches (low-carb eating, intermittent fasting, or a combination)
- Flexible and sustainable
- Focus on food quality and healthy fats
- Not obsessed with exact macronutrient ratios

"Keto Diet" (popular online version):

- Often rigid macronutrient ratios (75 percent fat, 20 percent protein, 5 percent carbs)
- Sometimes emphasizes processed "keto products" (bars, shakes, packaged foods)
- May prioritize ketone levels over overall health
- Can become obsessive and unsustainable
- Sometimes ignores food quality in favor of hitting macros

This chapter focuses on the principles of fat burning and metabolic flexibility, not rigid "keto" rules.

I'm not asking you to track every gram of fat, protein, and carbs. I'm not asking you to test your ketone levels obsessively. I'm simply showing you how to shift your metabolism toward fat burning by prioritizing healthy fats and strategically reducing carbohydrates.

Why Fat Became My Secret Weapon

For the first six months of my weight loss journey, I focused primarily on food order (Hack #1), low-glycemic swaps (Hack #2), and intermittent fasting (Hack #3). I was losing weight steadily and feeling good.

But I was still experiencing occasional cravings—especially in the evenings. I'd finish dinner satisfied, but two hours later, I'd find myself thinking about snacks. Ice cream. Chips. Something sweet or crunchy.

I wasn't giving in to these cravings most of the time, but the mental battle was exhausting. I was using willpower to resist, and willpower is a finite resource.

Then, I made a conscious decision to significantly increase my healthy fat intake while keeping my carb intake very low (under 50 grams per day).

Within three days, the cravings vanished. Completely.

It wasn't willpower. It wasn't discipline. My body stopped asking for those foods.

After dinner, I felt satisfied—genuinely, delighted—in a way I hadn't experienced in years. I could sit on the couch watching TV while my kids ate popcorn, and I had zero desire to join them. Not because I was "being good," but because I genuinely didn't want it.

That's when I understood the power of fat.

Fat provides satiety in a way that carbohydrates never can. Fat stabilizes your blood sugar. Fat keeps insulin low, which allows your body to access stored fat for energy. And when your body is efficiently burning fat for fuel, it doesn't send desperate hunger signals.

For many people, ketosis can dramatically reduce or eliminate cravings. For me, it was like someone turned off the hunger switch in my brain.

The Science: Why Fat Doesn't Make You Fat

Let's address the elephant in the room: If I'm eating more fat, won't I get fatter?

It's a logical question, given decades of "low-fat" diet advice. But in truth, healthy fats have a minimal impact on insulin levels compared to carbohydrates.

Remember, insulin is the hormone that determines whether your body stores fat or burns it. When insulin is high, you're in fat-storage mode. When insulin is low, you're in fat-burning mode.

What spikes insulin:

- Carbohydrates (especially refined carbs and sugar) → Major insulin spike
- Protein (moderate amounts) → Modest insulin response
- Fat → Minimal to no insulin response

Eating fat doesn't trigger the hormonal cascade that locks your body into fat-storage mode. Eating carbs does.

So when you eat fat in the absence of high carbohydrate intake, your body can use that fat for immediate energy without storing it. And when you're not eating (during fasting windows), your body can efficiently access stored body fat for fuel.

It may sound counterintuitive, but eating more fat can help you burn more fat—as long as you're keeping carbs low and insulin stable.

My Personal Experience: Discovering Fat-Burning

Let me walk you through how I transitioned to a fat-burning metabolism and what changed.

Before: High-Carb, Low-Fat (My First 40 Years)

For most of my life, I followed conventional dietary wisdom:

- Breakfast: Cereal with skim milk, orange juice, toast
- Lunch: Sandwich on whole wheat bread, baked chips, diet soda
- Snack: Low-fat yogurt, granola bar
- Dinner: Pasta with marinara sauce, side salad with fat-free dressing
- Evening: Low-fat ice cream or pretzels

What I was eating: Probably 60-70 percent carbohydrates, 20 percent protein, 10-20 percent fat

How I felt:

- Hungry every two to three hours
- Energy crashes mid-afternoon
- Constant cravings for sweets and starches
- Never felt truly satisfied after meals
- Gained weight steadily over the years

After: High-Fat, Low-Carb with Intermittent Fasting

Once I understood the power of fat and ketosis, my diet shifted dramatically. I combined the high-fat approach with intermittent fasting, typically practicing 16:8 or One Meal A Day (OMAD), depending on my schedule and hunger levels.

WHAT I WAS EATING (MACRONUTRIENT BREAKDOWN):

Roughly:

- 60 to 70 percent fat (from olive oil, butter, avocado, nuts, fatty fish, fatty cuts of meat)
- 20 to 25 percent protein (from meat, fish, eggs, cheese)
- 10 to 15 percent carbs (mostly from non-starchy vegetables, occasional berries)

Total net carbs: Usually 20 to 30 grams per day

WHY THIS APPROACH WORKED:

1. Extended fat-burning. With 16 to 23 hours of fasting, my body spent most of the day in fat-burning mode.
2. Stable energy. No blood sugar spikes or crashes, just steady, reliable energy from fat metabolism.
3. Mental clarity. Ketones fueled my brain efficiently. I felt sharper and more focused than ever.
4. No hunger. I genuinely wasn't hungry during fasting periods. The high-fat meals kept me satisfied for hours, sometimes an entire day.
5. Simplicity. OMAD meant one meal to think about, plan, and prepare. Life became simpler.
6. Social flexibility. I could schedule my eating window around social events, family dinners, or work commitments.

The Moment I Knew It Was Working

About two weeks into eating this way, I was at a birthday party for one of my kids' friends. There was a table loaded with food: pizza, chips, cookies, cake, and soda. The old me would have been drawn to that table like a magnet, eating "just one slice" that inevitably turned into three and sneaking cookies when no one was looking.

But standing there that day, I looked at all that food and felt … nothing.

No desire. No temptation. No internal battle.

I was genuinely satisfied with my lunch (salad with chicken thighs and avocado). My blood sugar was stable. My insulin was low. My body was happily burning fat for fuel.

I didn't eat a single thing at that party—not because I was "being good" or exerting willpower, but because I didn't want any of it.

That's when I knew this isn't a diet. This is freedom.

The Healthy Fats That Changed My Life

Not all fats are created equal. Some fats are incredibly beneficial for weight loss, health, and satiety. Others are inflammatory, processed, and harmful.

Here's how to tell the difference:

✅ HEALTHY FATS (Prioritize These)

These are the fats I eat regularly and without reservation:

1. Avocados and Avocado Oil

Why they're amazing:

- Loaded with heart-healthy monounsaturated fats
- High in potassium (more than bananas)
- Creamy, satisfying texture
- Versatile—eat plain, in salads, as guacamole, or cooked

How I use them:

- Half an avocado on my salad every day
- Guacamole as a side dish
- Avocado oil for high-heat cooking (it has a high smoke point)

2. Olive Oil (Extra Virgin)

Why it's fantastic:

- Rich in monounsaturated fats and antioxidants
- Anti-inflammatory properties
- Extensive research supporting heart health benefits
- Delicious flavor

How I use it:

- Drizzle on salads (primary salad dressing)
- Drizzle on cooked vegetables
- Mix with balsamic vinegar for dipping
- Light sautéing (not high heat—it has a lower smoke point)

Pro tip: Buy high-quality extra virgin olive oil in dark bottles. Cheap olive oil is often adulterated with other oils.

3. Fatty Fish (Salmon, Mackerel, Sardines)

Why they're amazing:

- High in omega-3 fatty acids (EPA and DHA)
- Support brain health, reduce inflammation, support heart health
- Excellent source of protein

How I use them:

- Wild-caught salmon two to three times per week (grilled, baked, or pan-seared)
- Canned sardines as a quick snack or lunch
- Smoked salmon on occasion

4. Nuts and Seeds

Why they're amazing:

- Healthy fats plus protein and fiber
- Portable, convenient snacks
- Keep you full for hours
- Provide vitamins, minerals, and antioxidants

My favorites:

- Brazil Nuts (rich in selenium)
- Almonds (my go-to snack)
- Walnuts (highest in omega-3s)
- Macadamia nuts (highest in monounsaturated fat)
- Pecans
- Chia seeds and flaxseeds (added to salads or smoothies)
- Pumpkin seeds

How I use them:

- Handful as an afternoon snack (10 to 15 nuts)
- Sprinkled on salads for crunch
- Almond butter on celery sticks

Caution: Nuts are calorie-dense. A small handful (about one ounce) is plenty. Don't mindlessly eat from a large container.

5. Coconut Oil and MCT Oil

Why they're amazing:

- Medium-chain triglycerides (MCTs) are rapidly absorbed and can be converted to ketones quickly
- May support ketosis even with slightly higher carb intake
- Antimicrobial properties
- Stable at high heat (suitable for cooking)

How I use them:

- Coconut oil for cooking (especially for eggs or stir-fries)
- MCT oil in my coffee occasionally (though I prefer black coffee during fasting)

6. Grass-Fed Butter and Ghee

Why they're amazing:

- Rich, satisfying flavor
- Contains beneficial compounds like CLA (conjugated linoleic acid) and butyrate

- Grass-fed butter has better omega-3 to omega-6 ratio than conventional
- Ghee (clarified butter) is lactose-free and has a high smoke point

How I use them:

- Butter on vegetables (broccoli with butter is a staple)
- Cooking eggs and meats
- Ghee for high-heat cooking

Note: Yes, butter is a saturated fat. For decades, we were told that saturated fat is bad. Current research suggests the relationship is more nuanced—especially when saturated fat is consumed in the context of a low-carb, whole-foods diet. I eat butter regularly, and my health markers have improved dramatically since I started.

7. Eggs (Especially the Yolks)

Why they're amazing:

- Yolks contain most of the nutrients (vitamins A, D, E, K, B vitamins, choline)
- Healthy fats and high-quality protein
- Incredibly satiating
- Versatile and inexpensive

How I use them:

- Scrambled eggs with vegetables for lunch
- Hard-boiled eggs as snacks
- Omelets loaded with veggies and cheese

Myth-busting: Eggs don't cause high cholesterol. For most people, dietary cholesterol has little impact on blood cholesterol levels. I eat 6 to 10 eggs per week, and my cholesterol has improved.

8. Full-Fat Dairy (If Tolerated)

Why it's fantastic:

- More satisfying than low-fat versions
- Contains fat-soluble vitamins
- Lower insulin response than low-fat dairy (which often has added sugar)

What I eat:

- Full-fat Greek yogurt (unsweetened)
- Cheese (cheddar, mozzarella, parmesan, goat cheese)
- Heavy cream (small amounts in coffee on non-fasting days, or with berries)

Note: Some people don't tolerate dairy well. If you experience digestive issues, bloating, or skin problems, consider eliminating dairy for two to three weeks and see if symptoms improve.

✗ UNHEALTHY FATS (Minimize or Avoid)

1. Trans Fats (Avoid Completely)

Found in:

- Hydrogenated and partially hydrogenated oils
- Many processed baked goods (crackers, cookies, pastries)
- Margarine and shortening
- Some fried fast foods

Why they're terrible:

- Increase LDL („bad") cholesterol
- Decrease HDL („good") cholesterol
- Linked to heart disease, inflammation, and insulin resistance
- Banned or restricted in many countries

What to do: Read labels. If you see "partially hydrogenated oil," avoid it altogether.

2. Excessive Industrial Seed Oils/Vegetable Oils

Common ones:

- Soybean oil
- Corn oil
- Canola oil (in excess)
- Cottonseed oil
- Sunflower oil (in excess)
- Safflower oil (in excess)

Why they can be problematic:

- High in omega-6 fatty acids (modern diets have too much omega-6 relative to omega-3)
- Often highly processed using heat and chemicals
- Prone to oxidation (becoming rancid)
- May contribute to inflammation when consumed in large amounts

My approach: I don't obsess over eliminating these oils (they're everywhere in processed foods and restaurants), but I don't cook with them at home. I prioritize olive oil, avocado oil, coconut oil, and butter instead.

3. Rancid or Oxidized Fats

How fats go bad:

- Exposure to heat, light, and air causes oxidation
- Rancid fats taste off and can be harmful

How to prevent:

- Store oils in dark bottles in cool places
- Don't reuse cooking oil multiple times
- Smell oils before using—if they smell "off," discard them
- Buy smaller bottles of oil and use them within a few months

How to Transition to a Fat-Burning Metabolism

If you've been eating a high-carb diet your whole life, transitioning to fat-burning takes time. Your body needs to adapt. Here's how I did it:

Phase 1: Reduce Carbs Gradually (Weeks 1 to 2)

Don't go from 300g of carbs per day to 20g overnight. That's a recipe for misery.

What I did:

- Eliminated obvious sugars and refined carbs (soda, candy, pastries, white bread)
- Replaced high-carb foods with low-glycemic swaps (cauliflower rice instead of white rice, zucchini noodles instead of pasta)

- Still ate some carbs (sweet potatoes, berries, occasional quinoa), but reduced portions

Target: Aim for about 100 to 150g of carbs per day in this phase

Phase 2: Increase Healthy Fats (Weeks 2 to 4)

As you reduce carbs, you need to replace those calories with something. That something is healthy fats.

What I did:

- Added avocado to every salad
- Cooked vegetables in butter or olive oil
- Ate fatty cuts of meat (ribeye, chicken thighs with skin, salmon)
- Snacked on nuts instead of crackers or granola bars
- Used full-fat dairy instead of low-fat

Important: Don't fear fat. Your body needs fuel. If you cut carbs *and* keep fat low, you'll be starving and miserable.

Phase 3: Push Into Ketosis (Week 4+)

Once you're comfortable with lower carbs and higher fat, you can push into ketosis if you choose.

What I did:

- Reduced carbs to under 50g per day (some days under 30g)
- Kept protein moderate (not excessive—too much protein can be converted to glucose)
- Filled the rest with healthy fats
- Combined with intermittent fasting (16:8 or 18:6)

Within three to five days, I was in ketosis.

The "Keto Flu" (And How to Avoid It)

During the first three to seven days of transitioning to ketosis, many people experience what's called the "keto flu":

Symptoms:

- Fatigue or low energy
- Headaches
- Brain fog
- Irritability
- Mild nausea
- Muscle cramps

What's happening: Your body is switching fuel sources. Your brain is adapting to using ketones instead of glucose. You're also losing water weight rapidly (carbs hold water in your body), which can cause electrolyte imbalances.

How to minimize or avoid it:

1. Stay hydrated. Drink lots of water (10 or more glasses per day).
2. Add electrolytes. Increase salt intake (add salt to food, drink bone broth), eat potassium-rich foods (avocados, spinach), and consider a magnesium supplement.
3. Don't cut calories. Eat enough fat. You're not trying to starve; you're trying to adapt.
4. Be patient. The symptoms are temporary. Within a week, you'll feel better than ever.

5. Reduce exercise intensity. Go easy during the adaptation period. Walk instead of doing intense workouts.

My experience: I had mild headaches and fatigue for about four days. Then, on Day Five, I woke up feeling incredible—clear-headed, energized, and completely free of cravings. It was worth the brief discomfort.

Signs You're in Ketosis (Beyond Testing)

You don't need to obsess over ketone levels. Your body will tell you if you're in ketosis.

Positive Signs:

- ✅ Reduced hunger. Can easily go four to six (or more) hours without eating.
- ✅ Stable energy. No mid-afternoon crashes or energy spikes.
- ✅ Mental clarity and focus. Brain feels sharp, productive.
- ✅ Decreased sugar cravings. Sweets no longer appeal to you.
- ✅ Slight fruity smell to breathe. Acetone (a ketone) is released in the breath.
- ✅ Weight loss. Especially when combined with other hacks.
- ✅ Better sleep. Many people report improved sleep quality.

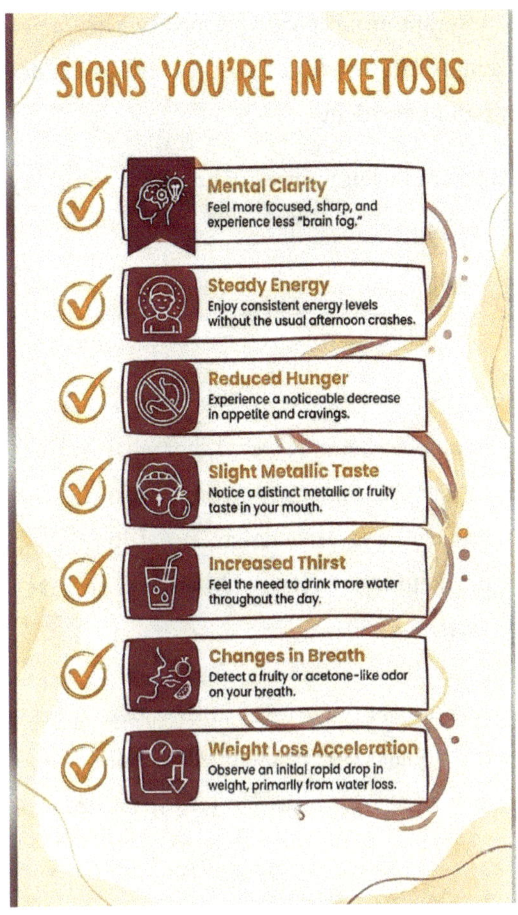

Initial Adaptation Signs (Temporary, Three to Seven days):

⚠ Mild fatigue or brain fog. The "keto flu" (can be easily managed with hydration and electrolytes).

⚠ Increased thirst. Your body is releasing water.

⚠ Changes in digestion. Bowel movements may change temporarily.

⚠ Slight irritability. Blood sugar regulation is adjusting.

These initial symptoms typically resolve within a week as your body fully adapts. Stay hydrated, add electrolytes (salt, potassium, magnesium), and be patient.

If symptoms persist beyond a week or are severe, consult your doctor.

Testing (Optional):

If you want to confirm ketosis, you can test ketone levels:

- Urine strips — Cheap, easy, but not very accurate (measures excess ketones being excreted, not what you're using).
- Blood ketone meter — More accurate, but strips are expensive (one to three dollars per strip).
- Breath ketone meter — Moderate accuracy, one-time purchase.

I tested occasionally out of curiosity at first, but I quickly learned to trust my body's signals. If I felt energized, clear-headed, and free of cravings, I knew I was in ketosis. No testing needed.

When Ketosis Isn't Right

Ketosis isn't for everyone, and that's perfectly okay. You can lose weight and improve health without ever entering ketosis.

Skip ketosis if:

- ❌ You're pregnant or breastfeeding.
- ❌ You have Type 1 diabetes.
- ❌ You have liver or pancreatic conditions.
- ❌ You have a history of eating disorders.

✗ You're a competitive athlete requiring high glycogen stores.

✗ You don't want to—and that's perfectly valid.

You can still use the other six hacks successfully without ketosis.

The low-glycemic swaps (Hack #2) naturally reduce carbs somewhat, but you don't need to go full ketogenic to see results. Many people lose significant weight and improve their health by eating 75 to 150g of carbs per day—nowhere near ketosis levels, but still much lower than the standard American diet.

The key principles apply regardless:

- Prioritize whole, unprocessed foods
- Choose healthy fats over unhealthy ones
- Keep insulin stable with food order and smart swaps
- Use intermittent fasting to give your body metabolic rest

These strategies work even if you never enter ketosis.

My Personal Approach: Flexible Fat-Burning

I want to be completely transparent about how I use ketosis in my life today, over a decade after starting this journey.

I don't live in strict ketosis 365 days a year. That would be unnecessarily rigid and unsustainable.

What I Do:

Most of the time (80 to 90 percent of days):

- Keep carbs relatively low (50 to 100g per day)

- Prioritize healthy fats at every meal
- Use intermittent fasting (16:8 or OMAD most days)
- My body is "fat-adapted"—comfortable and efficient at burning fat for fuel
- I'm likely in light ketosis or close to it most of the time

Sometimes (10 to 20 percent of days):

- Special occasions, holidays, vacations, celebrations
- I eat more carbs—pasta, bread, pizza, desserts
- I enjoy them thoroughly without guilt
- My body easily returns to fat-burning after one to two days

This flexibility is what makes it sustainable for life.

Rigid rules do not imprison me. I use ketosis as a tool, not a religion. When I want to tighten up (maybe I've been indulging more than usual), I can easily return to strict low-carb eating for a few days and drop right back into ketosis.

But most of the time, I'm simply eating real, whole foods with plenty of healthy fats, keeping carbs moderate, and letting my body do what it does naturally.

Practical Tips for Success with Healthy Fats

Here are the strategies that made this sustainable for me:

1. Cook Your Own Food

Restaurants and processed foods use cheap, unhealthy oils. When you cook at home, you control the quality of the fats you use.

What I do:

- Meal prep on Sundays (cook proteins, chop vegetables, portion snacks)
- Keep it simple—grilled meats, roasted vegetables, large salads
- Invest in good fats—quality olive oil, grass-fed butter, avocados

2. Always Have Healthy Fat Snacks Available

When hunger strikes, you'll reach for whatever's convenient. Make sure what's convenient is healthy.

What I keep on hand:

- Raw almonds, walnuts, and macadamia nuts in small containers
- Pre-portioned cheese cubes
- Hard-boiled eggs (make a batch weekly)
- Avocados (always have three to four ripe ones ready)
- Olives
- 85 percent dark chocolate (my evening treat)

3. Don't Fear Saturated Fat (In Context)

The old advice is that saturated fat causes heart disease. Avoid butter, red meat, and coconut oil.

The current understanding, however, is that saturated fat in the context of a low-carb, whole-foods diet doesn't appear to be harmful for most people. In fact, my cholesterol and heart health markers improved dramatically once I started eating butter and red meat regularly.

I eat saturated fats from whole food sources (butter, eggs, fatty meat, coconut oil) without fear. I balance them with plenty of monounsaturated fats (olive oil, avocados) and omega-3s (fish, walnuts).

Important caveat: This is for people following a low-carb diet. If you're eating high-carb and high-saturated-fat foods together, that's a different metabolic context. The combination of high carbs + high fat can be problematic.

4. The 85 percent Dark Chocolate Hack

For years, I'd eat milk chocolate or semi-sweet chocolate (50 to 60 percent cacao) and struggle to stop at just a square or two. The sugar content was high enough to trigger cravings for more.

Then I discovered 85 percent dark chocolate.

What's different:

- Very low sugar (usually five to eight grams per serving vs. 20 to 25g in milk chocolate)
- Rich, intense flavor—a little goes a long way
- High in antioxidants and beneficial compounds

My routine:

- Two squares after dinner
- Let it melt slowly on my tongue
- Deeply satisfying, no cravings for more

The first few times, 85 percent tastes bitter if you're used to sweeter chocolate. But within a week, your taste buds adapt. Now, milk chocolate tastes cloyingly sweet to me. I genuinely prefer 85 percent.

Tip: Start with 70 to 75 percent if 85 percent is too intense. Work your way up gradually.

5. Make Vegetables Delicious with Fat

One reason people fail at healthy eating is that they eat bland, steamed vegetables and hate them.

My solution: Make vegetables delicious with healthy fats.

Examples:

- Broccoli roasted in olive oil with salt and garlic
- Brussels sprouts cooked in bacon fat (yes, bacon fat)
- Spinach sautéed in butter with lemon
- Cauliflower mash with butter, cream, and parmesan
- Green beans with slivered almonds and olive oil

When vegetables taste amazing, you'll eat more of them. And that is ideal, because many vitamins (A, D, E, and K) are fat-soluble, meaning your body can only absorb them properly when consumed with fat.

6. Fat Coffee (If You Want)

Some people swear by adding butter and MCT oil to their coffee (often called "Bulletproof Coffee").

I prefer black coffee, but if you want to try it:

- 1 cup black coffee
- 1 tablespoon grass-fed butter or ghee
- 1 tablespoon MCT oil or coconut oil
- Blend until frothy

It's creamy, satisfying, may support ketosis, and keeps you full.

Caution: This breaks your fast (it contains calories). Use it during your eating window, not during fasting.

Common Mistakes with Healthy Fats and Ketosis

No matter how motivated you are, obstacles will arise. Here are the mistakes I see (and made myself):

Mistake #1: Not Eating Enough Fat

Cutting carbs while keeping fat low will leave you hungry, miserable, and low on energy.

Fat is your primary fuel source in ketosis. If you don't eat enough fat, you'll feel terrible—low energy, weak, irritable. Your body needs adequate fat to function optimally and maintain your metabolism. Too little fat can lead to metabolic slowdown over time.

When you cut carbs, increase fat proportionally. Eat until satisfied. Don't fear fat.

Mistake #2: Eating Too Much Protein

Going overboard on protein (multiple protein shakes, huge steaks, protein bars) while trying to do keto can cause the protein to be converted to glucose through gluconeogenesis, which can interfere with ketosis.

Keep protein moderate—about 20 to 25 percent of calories, or roughly 0.8 to 1.2g per kilogram of body weight. Prioritize fat, not protein, as your primary calorie source.

Mistake #3: Eating "Keto Junk Food"

Eating processed "keto" products (bars, cookies, ice cream) just because they're labeled "low-carb" or "keto" is not a good idea. Many of these products contain artificial sweeteners, unhealthy oils, and additives that can trigger cravings and inflammation.

Prioritize real, whole foods. If you want a treat, make it yourself with real ingredients (almond flour, coconut oil, 85 percent chocolate, etc.).

Mistake #4: Forgetting Vegetables

Eating bacon, butter, and steak without vegetables leads to digestive issues and nutrient deficiencies. You need the fiber, vitamins, minerals, and phytonutrients found in vegetables.

Half your plate should still be non-starchy vegetables, even on a high-fat diet. This is non-negotiable (see Hack #1!)

Mistake #5: Not Giving It Enough Time

Many try ketosis for three to four days, feel rough during the keto flu, and give up.

Adaptation takes at least a week or two. The first few days are the hardest. If you quit during the adaptation phase, you'll never experience the benefits.

Commit to at least two or three weeks. Push through the keto flu (stay hydrated, add salt). The benefits on the other side are worth it.

Mistake #6: Using Ketosis as an Excuse to Ignore Calories Completely

Don't start thinking to yourself, "I'm in ketosis, so I can eat unlimited amounts of fat and never gain weight!"

While ketosis makes it easier to naturally eat less (because fat is satiating), eating 4,000 calories a day will still prevent weight loss.

Let satiety guide you. Eat until satisfied (about 80 percent full), not stuffed. Trust that if you're eating real foods and honoring hunger signals, your body will regulate intake naturally.

Quick-Win Challenge: Your First Week of Fat-Burning

Ready to try the power of healthy fats? Here's your challenge:

Days 1 to 3: Add Healthy Fats, Reduce Sugar

Morning: Black coffee or tea

First Meal: Large salad with olive oil dressing, grilled chicken or salmon, half an avocado, a handful of nuts

Dinner: Fatty meat (ribeye, chicken thighs, pork chops) cooked in butter, roasted vegetables in olive oil, and a side of cauliflower mash

Snacks (if needed): Almonds, cheese, hard-boiled eggs

What to eliminate: All obvious sugars and refined carbs (soda, candy, pastries, white bread, pasta)

What to notice: How do you feel three to four hours after meals? Are you less hungry? More satisfied?

Days 4 to 7: Push Lower Carb

Continue above, but also:

- Reduce starchy vegetables (no potatoes, corn)
- Reduce fruit (berries only, small amounts)
- Increase fat at every meal
- Aim for under 50g of carbs per day

What to notice:

- Energy levels (may dip on days 4 and 5, then surge)
- Hunger (should decrease significantly)
- Cravings (should start to disappear)
- Mental clarity (should improve)

Stay hydrated. Add salt. Be patient.

End of Week Assessment:

Answer these questions:

1. How did I feel after eating more fat?
2. Did my hunger and cravings change?
3. Did I experience any keto flu symptoms?
4. Do I want to continue this approach?

If YES: Congratulations! You're on your way to fat-adaptation. If NO or "Not Sure": That's okay. You can still use moderate healthy fats and low-glycemic swaps without going full ketosis.

Why This Hack Is So Powerful

- ✅ It may dramatically reduce or eliminate cravings. Fat provides deep, lasting satiety.
- ✅ It can stabilize energy—no more blood sugar roller coaster.
- ✅ It keeps insulin low and allows your body to access stored fat for fuel.
- ✅ It supports brain health—your brain thrives on ketones.
- ✅ It improves metabolic flexibility. Your body becomes efficient at burning fat.
- ✅ It makes intermittent fasting easier. Fat-adapted people find fasting effortless.
- ✅ It transforms your relationship with food—food becomes fuel, not an obsession.

When I think back on my 80-pound weight loss, the shift to healthy fats and ketosis was the turning point. It's when weight loss went from "hard work requiring constant willpower" to "natural and almost effortless."

My body finally had the fuel it was designed to use. And once I unlocked that, everything else fell into place.

What's Next?

You now understand the power of healthy fats and how ketosis can transform your metabolism and eliminate cravings.

But even the best dietary strategies need practical support. That's where meal planning, grocery shopping, and food preparation come in.

In Chapter 8, you'll discover The Real Food Revolution—my strategies for meal prep, smart shopping, and building a sustainable food routine that fits into real life.

HACK #6—THE SCIENCE BEHIND MEAL PREP AND REAL FOOD

You can know everything about insulin, ketosis, food order, and intermittent fasting—but if you don't have a practical system for actually getting healthy food into your life, none of it matters.

This is where most diet books fail. They give you the theory, the science, and the inspiration, then leave you standing in your kitchen thinking, "Okay, so ... what do I actually eat? When do I shop? How do I prepare it? What if I don't have time?"

Hack #6 includes my proven strategies for meal prep, smart shopping, and building a sustainable food routine that fits into real life.

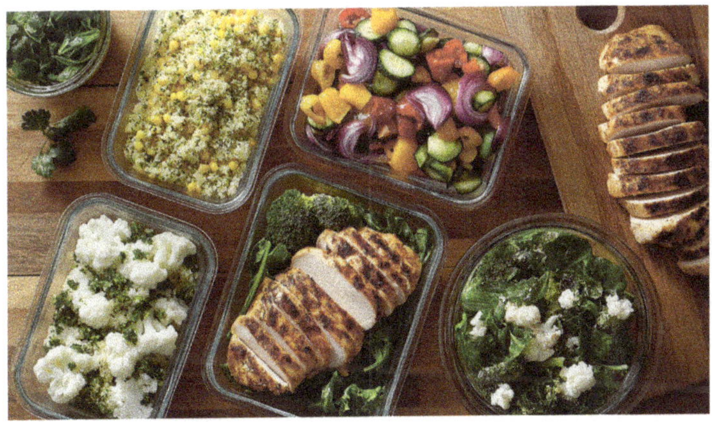

In this chapter, you'll discover my 90-minute Sunday meal prep routine that feeds me all week, along with precisely what to buy at the grocery store and what to avoid. You'll also learn simple and delicious recipes that support fat-burning, how to navigate restaurants without sabotaging your progress, and the systems that make healthy eating effortless, not exhausting.

Real food. Real life. Real results.

Let's make this practical.

The Sunday That Changed Everything

About four months into my weight loss journey, I had a problem.

My Monday through Friday mornings were going great. I'd wake up, do my seven-minute Tabata, drink black coffee, work all morning, then eat my first meal around noon—usually a big salad with grilled chicken, avocado, and olive oil.

But then the afternoon chaos would hit. Work deadlines. Kids' activities. Life. By 6 p.m., I'd be starving, exhausted, and standing in front of an empty fridge with no energy to cook.

That's when the dangerous thoughts would creep in: *Maybe I'll grab takeout ... just this once ... I've been good all week ...*

And before I knew it, I'd be eating pizza or Chinese food and undoing days of progress.

The problem wasn't willpower. The problem was a lack of preparation.

I was trying to make healthy choices when I was tired, hungry, and decision-fatigued. That's a recipe for failure.

So I decided to dedicate 90 minutes every Sunday to preparing food for the entire week.

That one change—spending 90 minutes on Sunday afternoon cooking and prepping—eliminated 90 percent of my weekday food stress.

Suddenly, healthy eating wasn't a constant battle—it was automatic. When I opened the fridge, nutritious food was right there, ready to eat.

The Real Food Revolution

Preparing your own meals from whole foods makes such a dramatic difference because while ultra-processed foods are engineered to override your body's natural satiety signals, real food works *with* your biology, not against it.

The Satiety Signal Hijack

Your body has sophisticated hunger and fullness sensors—hormones like leptin, ghrelin, and peptide tell your brain when you've had enough to eat. These sensors work perfectly when you eat real, whole foods that humans have eaten for millennia.

But ultra-processed foods are different. They're engineered in laboratories to hit the "bliss point"—the perfect combination of sugar, fat, salt, and texture that overrides your satiety signals. They're designed to make you eat more, not less. Food scientists call this "passive overconsumption"—you keep eating even when you're not hungry because the food hijacks your brain's reward system.

When you prepare meals from real, whole ingredients, something powerful kicks in: your body's natural hunger and fullness signals work correctly again. You eat when you're hungry. You stop when you're satisfied. You don't experience the intense cravings and loss of control that come from processed foods.

Without real food preparation, you're constantly battling food that's been engineered to make you overeat—and willpower alone can't win that fight.

The Research That Proves It Works

Multiple studies have confirmed the power of real food and home cooking:

Study 1: Ultra-Processed Foods Cause Overeating

A groundbreaking randomized controlled trial by Dr. Kevin Hall, published in *Cell Metabolism*, compared ultra-processed foods with whole foods in a controlled setting. Participants were given either ultra-processed meals or whole-food meals for two weeks, then switched. The results were shocking: when eating ultra-processed foods, people consumed an average of 500 more calories per day and gained 2 pounds—even though both diets had identical calorie, sugar, fat, fiber, and macronutrient content. The study proved that food processing itself—not just nutrients—drives overeating and weight gain.

Study 2: The NOVA Classification System

Research compiled by Dr. Carlos Monteiro and colleagues established the NOVA classification system, which categorizes foods by their degree of processing. Studies using this system found that ultra-processed foods now make up 60 percent of calories in the American diet—and every 10 percent increase in ultra-processed food consumption is associated with higher rates of obesity, Type 2 diabetes, cardiovascular disease, and even cancer. The research demonstrated that the rise in obesity parallels the rise in food processing, not just increased calorie availability.

Study 3: Home Cooking and Diet Quality

A study published in *Public Health Nutrition* examined the relationship between cooking at home and diet quality. The findings were clear: people who cooked at home more frequently consumed more fruits, vegetables, and whole foods, and less sugar, fat, and processed foods. Home cooking was associated with better diet quality regardless of income, education, or time availability. The researchers concluded that cooking is a critical life skill for health, not just a hobby for food enthusiasts.

Study 4: Long-Term Weight Gain and Food Choices

A landmark 20-year study published in the *New England Journal of Medicine* tracked over 120,000 health professionals and examined which specific foods were associated with weight gain or loss over time. The results were striking: the most significant contributors to weight gain were potato chips, potatoes, sugar-sweetened beverages, processed meats, and refined grains. The foods most associated with weight loss were vegetables, whole grains, fruits, nuts, and yogurt. The study showed that food quality matters more than calorie quantity—eating more of the right foods actually promotes weight loss.

Study 5: Satiety and Food Structure

Research on satiety has shown that whole foods with intact fiber, protein, and water content trigger fullness signals far more effectively than processed foods. Studies demonstrate that when you eat an apple (whole food), you feel satisfied and stop eating. But when you drink apple juice (processed, fiber removed), you consume far more calories without feeling full—and often continue eating other foods—the physical structure of food matters for satiety, not just its nutrient composition.

The science is precise: real food prepared at home restores your body's natural ability to regulate hunger and fullness—while ultra-processed foods are engineered to make you overeat.

Let me show you exactly how I do it.

My 90-Minute Sunday Meal Prep Routine

Every Sunday afternoon (usually between 2 and 4 p.m.), I spend 90 minutes in the kitchen. This is my non-negotiable time. I protect it like I'd protect an important meeting.

Here's the exact routine:

STEP 1: Protein Prep (30 minutes)

I cook three or four different proteins that will last the week:

1. Grilled Chicken Thighs (or breasts)

- Two to three pounds
- Season with salt, pepper, garlic powder, and paprika

- Grill or bake at 400°F (200°C) for 25 to 30 minutes
- Let cool, portion into containers (four to five servings)

2. Ground Beef or Turkey

- Two pounds
- Brown in a large skillet with onions and garlic
- Season with cumin, chili powder, salt
- Portion into containers (great for salads, lettuce wraps, or eggs)

3. Hard-Boiled Eggs

- 12 eggs
- Boil for 10 minutes, ice bath, peel
- Store in a container (perfect snacks or salad toppings)

4. Baked Salmon (optional)

- 1 to 1.5 pounds
- Season with lemon, dill, salt, olive oil
- Bake at 375°F (190°C) for 15 to 20 minutes
- Portion into containers (two to three servings)

Pro tip: I often rotate proteins week to week so I don't get bored. Some weeks it's steak. Some weeks, it's rotisserie chicken from the store (even easier). The key is variety and having it ready.

STEP 2: Vegetable Prep (30 minutes)

I prepare vegetables that can be eaten raw or quickly cooked:

What I prep:

1. Salad Base

- Wash and dry mixed greens, spinach, or romaine (enough for five to six large salads)
- Store in containers lined with paper towels to absorb moisture

2. Chopped Raw Vegetables

- Bell peppers (sliced)
- Cucumbers (sliced)
- Celery (cut into sticks)
- Cherry tomatoes (washed)
- Carrots (peeled and cut into sticks)
- Store in separate containers

3. Roasted Vegetables

- Broccoli florets
- Cauliflower florets
- Brussels sprouts (halved)
- Zucchini (sliced)

Toss with olive oil, salt, and garlic, spread on baking sheets, and roast at 425°F (220°C) for 20-25 minutes. Let cool, store in containers.

4. Cauliflower Rice

- Two to three bags of pre-riced cauliflower (or make your own)
- Sauté in butter or olive oil with garlic for five to seven minutes
- Portion into containers (perfect side dish all week)

STEP 3: Healthy Fats and Extras (15 minutes)

I prepare grab-and-go fat sources and flavor boosters:

What I prep:

1. Portioned Nuts

- Almonds, walnuts, or macadamia nuts
- Portion into small containers or bags (one ounce each = about 10 to 15 nuts)
- Grab-and-go snacks

2. Avocados

- Buy six or seven at various stages of ripeness (some ripe now, some for later in the week)
- No prep needed—have them ready

3. Homemade Salad Dressing

- Mix olive oil, balsamic vinegar, Dijon mustard, lemon juice, salt, pepper, and garlic
- Store in a jar (lasts all week)

4. Hard Cheese Cubes

- Cheddar, goat cheese, or parmesan
- Cut into cubes, store in a container
- Easy snacks

5. Fresh Herbs (if using)

- Wash and chop cilantro, parsley, or basil
- Store in a damp paper towel in a container

STEP 4: Assembly and Storage (15 minutes)

Now I organize everything in my fridge strategically:

- Top Shelf: Ready-to-eat proteins in clear containers (chicken, beef, salmon, eggs)
- Middle Shelf: Prepped vegetables in clear containers (salad greens, raw veggies, roasted veggies, cauliflower rice)
- Bottom Shelf: Fats and extras (nuts, cheese, avocados, dressing)
- Door: Condiments, olive oil, butter

Everything visible, everything accessible. No digging, no guessing. I can see at a glance what I have and what I need.

Total Time: 90 Minutes

What I've accomplished:

- Four or five days of lunch proteins ✅
- Five or six large salads ready to assemble ✅
- Roasted vegetables for dinners ✅
- Cauliflower rice sides ✅
- Grab-and-go snacks portioned ✅
- Dressing made ✅

What this means for my week:

- Lunch takes two minutes to assemble (grab a container of greens, add protein, drizzle dressing, add avocado)
- Dinner takes 10 minutes (reheat protein, reheat vegetables, done)
- Snacks are pre-portioned and ready
- Zero stress, zero decisions, zero excuses

Adapting Meal Prep to Your Life

My 90-minute Sunday routine works for me, but your situation may be different. Here's how to adapt:

If You Have a Large Family:

- Double or triple batch sizes
- Get family members involved (kids can wash vegetables, portion snacks, stir pots)
- Consider doing prep twice a week (Sunday and Wednesday) for maximum freshness
- Prep "components" rather than full meals—let family members customize their own plates

If You Live Alone:

- Cut the recipe sizes in half
- Focus on two or three proteins instead of four
- Consider freezing half of what you cook for the following week
- Meal prep might take you only 45 to 60 minutes

If You Have Limited Kitchen Space/Equipment:

- You don't need fancy equipment—a good knife, cutting board, one large skillet, and one baking sheet are sufficient
- Use your oven efficiently: roast vegetables on one sheet, protein on another, both at the same temperature
- One-pot meals work great (stews, chilis, stir-fries)

If You Work Weekends:

- Shift your prep day to whenever you have time—Wednesday evening, Monday morning, doesn't matter
- Or split it: 45 minutes twice a week instead of 90 minutes once

If You Hate Cooking:

- Keep it simple: rotisserie chicken from the store, pre-washed salad greens, canned fish, pre-cut vegetables
- You can "meal prep" by simply buying prepared healthy foods and portioning them
- Focus on assembly, not cooking

The principle remains the same: Dedicate focused time, once or twice a week, to preparing food. Make it a non-negotiable appointment with yourself. Protect it. Honor it.

Simple, Delicious Recipes

You don't need to be a chef to eat well. Here are my go-to meals—simple, fast, and delicious.

RECIPE 1: The Perfect Salad (My Daily Lunch)

Ingredients:

- 2 to 3 cups mixed greens or spinach
- 4 to 6 oz grilled chicken, salmon, or ground beef
- 1/2 avocado, sliced
- Handful of cherry tomatoes
- Sliced cucumber

- Handful of nuts (almonds or walnuts)
- Olive oil and balsamic vinegar (or lemon juice)
- Salt and pepper

Instructions:

1. Place greens in a large bowl
2. Add all toppings
3. Drizzle with olive oil and vinegar
4. Toss and enjoy

Time: two minutes (when ingredients are prepped)

Why it works: High in healthy fats, moderate protein, loaded with vegetables, minimal carbs, incredibly satisfying.

RECIPE 2: Cauliflower Fried "Rice"

Ingredients:

- 1 bag riced cauliflower (or 1 head cauliflower, riced in a food processor)
- 2 tablespoons butter or coconut oil
- 2 to 3 eggs, beaten
- 1/2 cup diced vegetables (bell peppers, peas, carrots)
- 2 cloves garlic, minced
- 2 tablespoons soy sauce or coconut aminos
- Green onions, sliced (optional)
- Cooked protein (chicken, shrimp, or beef)

Instructions:

1. Heat oil in a large skillet or wok over medium-high heat
2. Sauté garlic and vegetables for 2 to 3 minutes
3. Add cauliflower rice, stir-fry for 5 to 7 minutes until tender
4. Push the cauliflower to the side, and scramble eggs in the pan
5. Mix everything, add soy sauce, and stir
6. Top with cooked protein and green onions

Time: 15 minutes

Why it works: Tastes like fried rice but with 90 percent fewer carbs. Satisfying, flavorful, and filling.

RECIPE 3: Low-Carb Noodles with Meat Sauce

INGREDIENTS:

For the Meat Sauce:

- 1 pound ground beef or turkey
- 1 jar marinara sauce (check label—choose one with no added sugar)
- 2 cloves garlic, minced
- 1 tablespoon olive oil
- Italian seasoning, salt, pepper to taste
- Parmesan cheese (optional, for topping)

For the Noodles:

- Option A: Shirataki noodles or rice (1 bag) —Zero carbs, pre-packaged

- Option B: Zucchini noodles/zoodles (3 to 4 medium zucchini, spiralized, or buy 2 pre-spiralized bags) —Low-carb, fresh vegetable
  - 1 tablespoon olive oil is needed for the zucchini option

INSTRUCTIONS:

Step 1: Prepare Your Noodles

If using Shirataki noodles/rice:

1. Rinse thoroughly under cold water to remove the natural odor
2. Set aside (they'll be added directly to the warm sauce later)

If using zucchini noodles:

1. Heat 1 tablespoon olive oil in a separate pan over medium heat
2. Sauté zucchini noodles for 2 to 3 minutes only (don't overcook or they'll get mushy and watery)
3. Remove from heat and set aside

Step 2: Make the Meat Sauce

1. Heat a large skillet over medium-high heat
2. Add ground beef or turkey and minced garlic
3. Brown the meat, breaking it up as it cooks (about 5 to 7 minutes)
4. Drain excess fat if desired
5. Add marinara sauce and Italian seasoning, salt, and pepper
6. Simmer for 10 minutes, stirring occasionally

Step 3: Combine and Serve

If using Shirataki noodles/rice:

- Add the rinsed Shirataki directly into the meat sauce
- Stir gently and let heat through for 2 to 3 minutes
- The noodles will absorb the sauce flavors

If using zucchini noodles:

- Plate the sautéed zucchini noodles
- Top generously with the meat sauce
- (Don't mix zoodles into the sauce or they'll release water and become soggy)

Step 4: Finishing Touch

- Sprinkle with freshly grated Parmesan cheese if desired
- Add fresh basil or extra Italian seasoning for more flavor

CHEF'S NOTES:

Shirataki: Best for absorbing sauce, zero carbs, slightly chewy texture. My go-to for easy meal prep.

Zucchini: Fresh vegetable option, slight crunch, naturally sweet. Great if you prefer a lighter, veggie-forward dish.

Both work beautifully—choose whichever you prefer and what you have on hand!

Time: 30 minutes

Why it works: Pasta comfort food without the insulin spike, the meat sauce is so flavorful that you won't miss traditional pasta.

RECIPE 4: Simple Baked Salmon

Ingredients:

- 1 salmon fillet (6 to 8 oz)
- 1 tablespoon olive oil or butter
- Lemon juice
- Fresh dill or dried herbs
- Salt and pepper

Instructions:

1. Preheat oven to 375°F (190°C)
2. Place salmon on a baking sheet lined with parchment paper
3. Drizzle with olive oil, lemon juice, and sprinkle with herbs, salt, and pepper
4. Bake for 15 to 20 minutes (until salmon flakes easily with a fork)
5. Serve with roasted vegetables or cauliflower rice

Time: 20 minutes

Why it works: Minimal effort, maximum omega-3s and healthy fats, incredibly satisfying.

RECIPE 5: Egg and Vegetable Scramble

Ingredients:

- 3 eggs
- 1 tablespoon butter or coconut oil
- 1 cup chopped vegetables (spinach, bell peppers, mushrooms, onions)
- 1/4 avocado, sliced
- Salt, pepper, hot sauce (optional)
- Cheese (optional)

Instructions:

1. Heat butter in a skillet over medium heat
2. Sauté vegetables for 3 to 4 minutes until softened
3. Beat eggs, pour into skillet
4. Scramble until cooked to your preference
5. Plate, top with avocado slices, cheese if desired

Time: 10 minutes

Why it works: Perfect for breaking your fast, high in protein and healthy fats, loaded with vegetables, it keeps you full for hours.

RECIPE 6: Lettuce Wrap Tacos

Ingredients:

- Large lettuce leaves (butter lettuce or romaine)
- 1 pound ground beef, turkey, or chicken
- Taco seasoning (or cumin, chili powder, garlic, salt)
- Toppings: avocado, salsa, cheese, sour cream (or Greek yogurt), cilantro, lime

Instructions:

1. Brown ground meat in a skillet
2. Add taco seasoning and a splash of water, and simmer for 5 minutes
3. Wash and separate lettuce leaves
4. Fill leaves with meat and desired toppings
5. Fold and enjoy like a taco

Time: 15 minutes

Why it works: All the flavor of tacos without the high-carb tortilla. Satisfying, fun to eat, and completely customizable.

RECIPE 7: Roasted Chicken Thighs with Vegetables

Ingredients:

- 4 chicken thighs (bone-in, skin-on for more fat and flavor)
- 2 cups broccoli florets
- 2 cups Brussels sprouts, halved
- 2 tablespoons olive oil or avocado oil
- Garlic powder, paprika, salt, pepper

Instructions:

1. Preheat oven to 425°F (220°C)
2. Place chicken thighs and vegetables on a large baking sheet
3. Drizzle everything with oil, season generously
4. Roast for 35 to 40 minutes (chicken should reach 165°F internal temp)
5. Serve immediately

Time: 45 minutes (mostly hands-off)

Why it works: One-pan meal, minimal cleanup, maximum flavor. The chicken fat renders and flavors the vegetables beautifully.

The Pattern You'll Notice

All these recipes are:

- Simple (five to 10 ingredients max)
- Fast (10 to 45 minutes, many are much quicker)

- Based on real, whole foods
- High in healthy fats
- Moderate in protein
- Low in carbs
- Delicious enough to eat regularly without getting bored

You don't need complicated recipes. You need reliable, simple meals you can make repeatedly without having to think.

Navigating Restaurants and Social Situations

You can't meal prep your entire life. Sometimes you eat out. Sometimes you attend parties, dinners, or celebrations. Here's how to navigate these situations without sabotaging your progress.

Restaurant Strategy 1: Choose the Right Restaurant

Best choices:

- Steakhouses (grilled meat, side salads, vegetables)
- Seafood restaurants (fish, salads, non-starchy vegetables)
- Mexican restaurants (fajitas, lettuce-wrap tacos, guacamole)
- Mediterranean/Greek restaurants (grilled meats, olive oil, salads, hummus)

More challenging:

- Pasta-focused Italian restaurants
- Asian restaurants with heavy rice/noodle emphasis
- Fast food (though some have salad options)

When choosing where to eat, I gently steer the group toward restaurants I know have good options. If I can't decide, I adapt (see strategies below).

Restaurant Strategy 2: Modify Your Order

Most restaurants are happy to accommodate modifications. Don't be shy about asking.

What I say:

- "Can I substitute the rice/potatoes for extra vegetables?"
- "Could you prepare that grilled instead of fried?"
- „No bread basket, please."
- "Dressing on the side, please."
- "Can I get that without the bun/tortilla?"

Most servers are accommodating. You're not being difficult—you're being clear about what you want. And you're often paying the same price for a healthier meal.

Restaurant Strategy 3: Focus on What You CAN Eat

Instead of feeling deprived about what you're avoiding, focus on enjoying what you are eating:

- Perfectly grilled steak with compound butter
- Fresh fish with olive oil and lemon
- Large salad with real olive oil dressing
- Avocado (many restaurants will add it to anything)
- Sautéed vegetables in butter
- Cheese, olives, nuts as appetizers

Restaurant meals can be absolutely delicious when you focus on high-quality proteins, fats, and vegetables. You're not suffering—you're eating well.

Restaurant Strategy 4: Skip the Alcohol (Or Choose Wisely)

Alcohol has two problems:

1. It contains calories (often significant)
2. It lowers inhibitions, making you more likely to overeat or make poor food choices

My approach:

- I rarely drink alcohol (maybe a few times per year)
- When I do, I choose dry red wine or spirits with soda water (no sugary mixers)
- I never drink on an empty stomach
- I limit myself to one drink

If you choose not to drink, order sparkling water with lime. No one cares, and you'll feel better the next day.

Social Situation Strategy: Parties and Gatherings

The challenge: Tables loaded with chips, crackers, cookies, cake, soda. Social pressure to "just have a little."

My strategies:

1. Eat Before You Go

- Have a satisfying meal (protein, fat, vegetables) before attending
- You'll arrive full, making it much easier to resist temptations

2. Bring a Healthy Dish

- Bring a veggie tray with guacamole
- Bring a cheese and nut platter
- Bring deviled eggs
- This ensures there's at least one thing you can eat

3. Position Yourself Away From Food

- Don't stand next to the snack table
- Engage in conversations away from the food area
- Out of sight, out of mind

4. Hold a Drink

- Sparkling water, unsweetened iced tea, or even just water in a nice glass
- Having something in your hand reduces the urge to grab food

5. Be Honest (If Asked)

- "I'm not eating that right now—I'm focusing on feeling my best."
- "I already ate, but thank you!"
- "This looks great, but no thank you. I'm good."

Most people don't care what you're eating. They're focused on themselves. And if someone does push ("Oh come on, just one bite!"). A polite but firm "No, thank you" is enough.

Common Obstacles and Solutions

Obstacle 1: "I Don't Have Time"

Reality check: You have time. You're just choosing to spend it on other things.

Solution:

- 90 minutes once a week is 1.2 percent of your week
- Most people spend more time than that scrolling social media
- Meal prep saves time during the week (no daily cooking stress)
- It's an investment that pays dividends all week

Reframe: "I invest 90 minutes in meal prep because my future self thanks me for that every single day."

Obstacle 2: "I Don't Like Cooking"

Solution:

- You don't have to love cooking—you need to do basic preparation
- Keep it simple: grilled chicken, roasted vegetables, salads
- Use shortcuts: rotisserie chicken, pre-cut vegetables, canned fish
- Think of it as "assembly", not "cooking"

Obstacle 3: "My Family Won't Eat This Way"

Solution:

- Cook the protein and vegetables the same for everyone
- Add rice/pasta as a side for family members who want it
- Many of these meals are customizable (like lettuce wrap tacos—give them tortillas, while you use lettuce)
- Lead by example: when they see your results and energy, they may become curious and want to try it themselves

Obstacle 4: "Healthy Food Is Boring"

Solution:

- Healthy food is only dull if you make it boring
- Use spices, herbs, and healthy fats generously
- Experiment with different cuisines
- Try new vegetables and proteins regularly
- Don't eat the same meal every day

Obstacle 5: "I Travel a Lot for Work"

Solution:

- Pack portable snacks: nuts, cheese, hard-boiled eggs, dark chocolate
- Choose hotels with mini-fridges (store your own food)
- Research restaurants in advance (steakhouses, seafood, salad spots)
- Intermittent fasting makes travel easier (skip hotel breakfast, eat well at lunch/dinner)
- Many grocery stores have prepared options (rotisserie chicken, salad bars)

Obstacle 6: "It's More Expensive"

Solution:

- Compared to eating out or ordering delivery, home cooking is actually far cheaper
- Buy frozen vegetables (just as nutritious, less expensive)
- Eggs are an incredibly cheap source of protein
- Buy in bulk for non-perishables
- One $12 fast food meal = ingredients for two to three home-cooked meals

The real cost of not eating well is much higher: medical bills, medications, lost productivity, and lower quality of life. Investing in real food now saves money in the long term.

Quick-Win Challenge: Your First Meal Prep Sunday

Ready to try meal prep? Here's your simplified challenge for this week:

This Sunday: 60-Minute Beginner Meal Prep

You don't need to do everything I do. Start small.

What to prep:

1. One protein (20 minutes)

- Grill or bake chicken breasts or thighs
- Or buy a rotisserie chicken and shred it
- Portion into four containers

2. One vegetable (20 minutes)

- Roast broccoli and cauliflower (toss with olive oil, salt, and roast at 425°F for 20 minutes)
- Portion into four containers

3. Salad base (10 minutes)

- Wash and dry mixed greens
- Store in a large container with a paper towel

4. Snacks (10 minutes)

- Portion five to six small bags of almonds (one ounce each)
- Hard-boil six eggs

Total Time: 60 minutes

What you now have:

- Four easy lunches (salad + chicken + olive oil dressing)
- Four easy dinners (chicken + roasted vegetables)
- Snacks ready to grab

Next Week:

- Add one more protein
- Add one more vegetable
- Gradually build up to a complete 90-minute prep

The key: Start small, build momentum, make it a habit.

Why This Hack Is So Powerful

- ✓ Eliminate decision fatigue—no more "what should I eat?" stress.
- ✓ Remove temptation. Healthy food is ready; junk food isn't in the house.
- ✓ Save time during busy weekdays—two-minute lunch assembly vs. 30 minutes of cooking.
- ✓ Save money. Research from the U.S. Department of Agriculture found that meals prepared at home cost approximately 60 percent less per calorie than restaurant meals.
- ✓ Guarantee nutrition. You control ingredients, quality, and portions.
- ✓ Build sustainable habits—systems that work long-term, not systems reliant on short-term willpower.
- ✓ Make healthy eating automatic. The default choice becomes the healthy choice.

Looking back at my 80-pound weight loss, meal prep was the hidden MVP. It wasn't glamorous or exciting, but it was the practical system that made everything else possible.

You can know all the hacks in the world, but if you don't have healthy food on hand, you'll fail. Meal prep ensures you succeed.

What's Next?

You now have the practical systems for making healthy eating effortless: meal prep routines, shopping strategies, simple recipes, and restaurant navigation.

But all of this only works if you can sustain it for life. That's where the final hack comes in: The 80/20 Flexibility Principle.

CHAPTER 9

HACK #7—THE 80/20 FLEXIBILITY PRINCIPLE

You've learned six powerful hacks that address insulin resistance and create sustainable weight loss:

1. Food order (vegetables first)
2. Low-glycemic swaps
3. Intermittent fasting
4. Movement integration
5. Healthy fats and ketosis
6. Real food and meal prep

Each hack works. Each hack compounds with the others. Together, they create a comprehensive system for metabolic health.

But here's the problem with most health books: They assume you'll follow the rules perfectly, forever.

They give you the strategies, then send you off with the implicit message: "Now do this 100 percent of the time, for the rest of your life."

And when you inevitably can't maintain perfection—because you're human, and life happens—you feel like you've failed. So you quit.

This is where most people lose the weight … and then gain it all back.

I know, because I almost made this mistake myself.

Important Medical Note: If you have diabetes (Type 1 or Type 2), pre-diabetes, or any metabolic condition requiring consistent carbohydrate intake, consult your healthcare provider before implementing flexible eating patterns. Blood sugar stability may require more consistency than the following 80/20 approach allows.

This chapter provides the author's experience, not medical advice.

My Dangerous Flirtation with Perfection

About eight months into my weight loss journey, I'd lost nearly 70 pounds. I was feeling incredible. My energy was through the roof. My clothes fit better than they have in years. People were constantly noticing and complimenting me.

I became rigid.

I followed the hacks perfectly—every single day. No exceptions.

- Vegetables first at every meal? Check.
- 16:8 fasting window? Never missed.
- No processed foods? Not even a bite.
- Exercise every morning? Rain or shine, no matter what.

I became proud of my discipline. I felt superior to my "old self," who couldn't control his eating. I started judging others who weren't as "committed" as I was.

And then came my daughter's birthday party.

The Birthday Cake That Almost Broke Me

When my youngest daughter turned seven, we had a small party at home—just family and a few of her friends. My wife ordered her favorite cake from the local bakery: chocolate with vanilla buttercream frosting.

When it was time to sing "Happy Birthday," everyone gathered around. Candles were lit. My daughter's face glowed with excitement.

She blew out the candles. Everyone clapped. Cake was served.

And I … stood there, arms crossed, refusing to eat any.

"No, thank you," I said when offered a slice. "I don't eat sugar."

My daughter looked at me with confusion. Then disappointment.

"Daddy, it's my birthday cake," she said quietly.

I held firm. "I know, honey. But Daddy doesn't eat cake anymore. It's not healthy."

She didn't say anything else. But I saw the hurt in her eyes.

Later that night, after the guests had left and the kids were in bed, my wife sat me down.

"You made your daughter feel bad on her birthday," she said gently.

"I didn't mean to," I defended. "I'm just trying to stay healthy. You know how hard I've worked—"

She interrupted. "You had a choice. You could have eaten one small slice of cake, celebrated with your daughter, and gone right back to your healthy habits the next day. Instead, you chose rigidity over a relationship."

That hit me hard.

She was right. In my quest for perfect adherence to my new lifestyle, I'd lost sight of what mattered most: being present with the people I love.

I'd turned healthy eating into an inflexible religion. And that rigidity wasn't sustainable—or even desirable.

That's when I realized I needed Hack #7.

What Is the 80/20 Principle?

The 80/20 Flexibility Principle is simple: follow your healthy habits 80 percent of the time. Be flexible and enjoy life 20 percent of the time.

This isn't about "cheat days" or "going off the wagon." It's about intentional flexibility that lets you maintain your results while still enjoying special moments, social events, and the foods you love.

The math:

- Seven days per week = 21 meals (assuming three meals/day, or two meals + snacks)
- 80 percent adherence = 17 meals, following your healthy habits
- 20 percent flexibility = four meals where you're more relaxed

Or, if you prefer to think weekly:

- Five to six days per week: Strict adherence to Hacks 1 through 6
- One or two days per week: Flexible meals or treats

The key: You're still following healthy principles *most of the time.* You're just allowing space for real life.

The Science Behind Flexibility and Sustainability

So why does allowing yourself 20 percent flexibility actually help you lose weight and keep it off? The answer lies in the psychology of restriction and how rigid dieting backfires by triggering binge eating and diet abandonment.

The Restriction-Binge Cycle

Think of willpower as a muscle that gets fatigued with constant use. When you follow an extremely rigid diet with zero flexibility—telling yourself you can "never" have certain foods—you're constantly flexing that willpower muscle. Eventually, it gives out.

What happens next is predictable: you break the rule. Maybe you eat a cookie. And because you've been in "all-or-nothing" mode, that single cookie triggers a psychological spiral: "I've already ruined everything, so I might as well eat the whole box." One slight deviation becomes a full-blown binge, followed by guilt, shame, and often complete diet abandonment.

But when you build flexibility into your approach—knowing that 20 percent of your meals can be imperfect without derailing your progress—the forbidden fruit loses its power. You can have a cookie, enjoy it, and move on. There's no spiral. No binge. No guilt. Just a regular part of sustainable eating.

Research shows that this flexible approach doesn't just work better psychologically—it also produces better long-term weight-loss results than rigid dieting.

The Research That Proves It Works

Multiple studies have confirmed the power of flexible eating strategies:

Study 1: Rigid vs. Flexible Dieting and Eating Disorders

A study published in the journal *Appetite* examined the relationship between dieting style and eating disorder symptoms in women. The findings were striking: rigid dietary control—having absolute rules about food—was strongly associated with binge eating, emotional eating, and eating disorder symptoms. In contrast, flexible dietary control—allowing occasional indulgences while maintaining overall healthy patterns—was associated with lower BMI, less binge eating, and better psychological outcomes. The researchers concluded that how you diet matters as much as what you eat.

Study 2: Flexible Control Predicts Long-Term Success

A study published in *Appetite* compared rigid and flexible dieting strategies and their relationship to weight outcomes. The study found that rigid dieters were more likely to experience mood disturbances, anxiety about eating, and episodes of overeating. Flexible dieters, on the other hand, maintained their weight loss more successfully and reported lower levels of depression and anxiety. The key difference: flexible dieters could adapt to real-life situations without feeling like failures, while rigid dieters spiraled when perfection became impossible.

Study 3: The Lean Habits Study—Three-Year Weight Maintenance

A landmark study published in the *International Journal of Obesity* followed successful weight-loss maintainers for 3 years to identify what separated those who kept weight off from those who regained it. The results were precise: flexible dietary control was one of the strongest predictors of long-term success. People who allowed themselves occasional treats while maintaining healthy overall eating patterns kept the weight off. Those who tried to maintain rigid control were more likely to regain weight. The study demonstrated that sustainability trumps perfection.

Study 4: Psychological Impact of Dietary Restraint

Research has shown that telling yourself you "can't" have certain foods actually increases cravings for those foods and makes you more likely to overeat them when willpower fails. This phenomenon, known as "ironic process theory" or the "forbidden fruit effect," demonstrates that restriction creates psychological reactance—a rebellious desire to do precisely what you've forbidden yourself from doing. Flexible approaches that allow occasional indulgences prevent this psychological backlash and make long-term adherence possible.

Study 5: Real-World Sustainability

Studies on long-term weight loss maintenance consistently show that the most successful maintainers don't follow perfect diets—they follow sustainable patterns that allow for flexibility, enjoyment, and social connection. Research from the *National Weight Control Registry*, which tracks over 10,000 people who've lost significant weight and kept it off, shows that successful maintainers don't deprive themselves of all treats. Instead, they practice consistent healthy eating most of the time while allowing room for life's celebrations and imperfections.

The science is precise: flexibility isn't weakness—it's the key to long-term success. The 80/20 approach works because it's sustainable, psychologically healthy, and aligned with how humans actually live.

Why 80/20 Works (And 100 percent Adherence Doesn't)

Reason #1: Sustainability

Perfection is not sustainable.

- You can white-knuckle your way through perfect adherence for weeks, maybe even months. But eventually, life happens. Weddings, holidays, vacations, stressful weeks—these moments make strict eating habits nearly impossible to maintain.

But if your approach to health doesn't allow for these moments, you'll either:

1. Miss out on life (like I almost did with my daughter's birthday)
2. Break your rules, feel guilty, and spiral into abandoning all your progress

The 80/20 Principle permits you to participate in life without guilt or self-sabotage.

Reason #2: Psychology of Restriction

Research in behavioral psychology consistently shows that the more you restrict something, the more you crave it.

When you tell yourself, "I can never have cake again," your brain becomes obsessed with cake. It's all you think about. Every birthday party, every bakery window, every dessert menu becomes a battle of willpower.

But when you tell yourself, *"I can have cake sometimes, when it's special,"* the urgency disappears.

You're not depriving yourself forever. You're just choosing when and how often to indulge. That psychological shift is decisive.

Reason #3: Metabolic Flexibility

Interestingly, occasional carb refeeds can actually benefit your metabolism, especially if you've been eating low-carb or keto for extended periods.

When you eat very low-carb for weeks or months, your body becomes incredibly efficient at burning fat. But some people experience:

- Thyroid hormone reduction (T3 levels drop slightly)
- Leptin reduction (the hormone that signals "I'm full")
- Cortisol elevation (from prolonged carb restriction stress)

Strategic carb refeeds—eating more carbs one or two times per week—can:

- Boost leptin levels (improving satiety signals)
- Support thyroid function
- Replenish glycogen stores (improving workout performance)
- Give you a psychological break from restriction

This isn't "cheating." It's metabolic flexibility—teaching your body to burn both fat and carbs efficiently.

Reason #4: Social Connection

Humans are social creatures, and food is deeply tied to connection, celebration, and culture.

When you rigidly refuse to participate in food-centered social events, you risk isolating yourself.

You become "that person" who can't eat at restaurants, who brings their own food to parties, who makes everyone uncomfortable with their restrictions.

The 80/20 Principle allows you to:

- Share meals with friends and family
- Celebrate special occasions without stress
- Travel and experience new cuisines
- Maintain relationships without food becoming an obstacle

Your health matters, but so do your relationships.

The Rules of Flexibility

Flexibility doesn't mean chaos. It means intentional, planned enjoyment without guilt.

Here are the rules I follow:

Rule #1: Flexibility is Planned, Not Impulsive

❌ DON'T: Decide randomly, "I feel like having pizza tonight," when you're stressed or bored.

✅ DO: Plan. "This Saturday is date night with my wife. We're going to our favorite Italian restaurant, and I'm going to enjoy pasta and wine."

Impulsive flexibility often leads to emotional eating, guilt, and spiraling. Planned flexibility, meanwhile, is a conscious choice—you enjoy it thoroughly, without regret, and return to healthy habits immediately after.

Rule #2: Ask "Is This Special?"

Not every treat deserves your 20 percent.

Before indulging, ask yourself: "Is this special, or is it just available?"

Examples:

Special:

- Your daughter's birthday cake (served with love, once a year)
- A meal at a Michelin-star restaurant on vacation
- Your grandmother's homemade lasagna at Thanksgiving
- Champagne at your best friend's wedding

Just Available:

- Gas station donuts
- Break room birthday cake for someone you barely know
- Grocery store cookies on sale
- Drive-thru fast food because it's convenient

Save your flexibility for what truly matters. Don't waste it on mediocre, convenient junk.

Rule #3: Enjoy It Fully, Without Guilt

When you choose to be flexible, commit to enjoying it.

Don't eat the birthday cake while thinking, "This is so bad. I'm ruining everything. I shouldn't be doing this." That guilt destroys the psychological benefit of flexibility and makes you more likely to spiral.

Instead, eat the cake slowly. Savor every bite. Enjoy the moment with your daughter. Then move on.

No guilt. No shame. Just a conscious choice, thoroughly enjoyed. Then, jump back to healthy habits.

Rule #4: Return to 80 percent immediately.

This is the most important rule.

Flexibility becomes destructive when one flexible meal turns into a flexible day, which turns into a flexible week, which turns into abandoning all progress.

The solution: Return to your healthy habits at the very next meal.

Example:

- Saturday night: You enjoy pizza and dessert at a dinner party
- Sunday morning: You're back to your routine—intermittent fasting, vegetables first, low-glycemic foods

No "I already ruined the weekend, might as well keep going" mentality.

One flexible meal doesn't erase weeks of progress. But a week of flexible meals can.

Rule #5: Track Your Balance

It's easy to think you're following 80/20 when you're actually closer to 60/40 or even 50/50.

How to track:

At the end of each week, count your meals:

- How many meals followed the hacks?
- How many were flexible?

If you're consistently below 80 percent, your results will stall. If you're consistently at 90 to 95 percent, you might be too rigid and headed for burnout.

80/20 is the sweet spot.

What 80/20 Looks Like in Real Life

Let me show you how I apply this principle across different scenarios.

A Typical Week for Me:

Monday-Friday:

- 16:8 intermittent fasting or OMAD
- Vegetables first at every meal
- Low-glycemic foods
- Healthy fats and protein
- Meal-prepped lunches and dinners
- Seven-minute morning Tabata

Saturday:

- Morning: Normal routine (fasting, Tabata)
- Lunch: Normal meal (vegetables first, protein, healthy fats)
- Evening: Date night with my wife—flexible meal. We go to a nice restaurant. I order what sounds good, including a glass of wine and maybe dessert. I enjoy it thoroughly, no guilt.

Sunday:

- Back to routine immediately
- Intermittent fasting
- Healthy meals
- Movement

Total flexibility: one flexible meal out of 14 to 16 meals = ~six to seven percent flexibility.

But some weeks, I have more. If there's a holiday, a vacation, or multiple social events, I might have two or three flexible meals in a week. That's still only ~15-20 percent flexibility.

The key: I'm intentional. I plan it. I enjoy it. And I return to healthy habits immediately.

Social Situations Made Simple

One of the biggest challenges in maintaining weight loss is navigating social situations where food plays a central role. Chapter 10 covers detailed strategies for handling these scenarios long-term, but the 80/20 principle makes them simple:

The core approach:

- Plan your flexibility around truly special occasions
- Follow the "Is this special?" guideline
- Enjoy without guilt when you choose to indulge
- Return to 80 percent immediately after

That's it. You'll learn specific tactics for restaurants, holidays, and travel in the next chapter, but remember: 80/20 permits you to participate in life while maintaining your results.

When Your Identity Changes, Everything Else Follows

When your identity shifts from "person trying to lose weight" to "healthy person who makes good choices," flexibility becomes natural.

A healthy person eats cake at their daughter's birthday—because that's what loving parents do.

A healthy person enjoys wine and pasta on vacation—because experiencing life entirely is part of being healthy.

A healthy person returns to vegetables, protein, and fasting the next day—because that's who they are.

You're not "cheating" or "being bad" when you're flexible. You're being a well-rounded human who prioritizes both health and relationships.

How to Know If You're Doing 80/20 Right

Signs you're doing it well:

- ✅ You enjoy flexible meals without guilt.
- ✅ You return to healthy habits immediately after.
- ✅ Your weight stays stable or continues to drop slowly.
- ✅ You don't feel deprived or restricted.
- ✅ You can navigate social situations without stress.
- ✅ You're maintaining your results for months, not just weeks.
- ✅ Food doesn't constantly dominate your thoughts.

Signs you're being too rigid (not enough flexibility):

- ⚠️ You avoid social events because of food
- ⚠️ You feel anxious or guilty about every food choice
- ⚠️ You think about food constantly
- ⚠️ You can't remember the last time you enjoyed a meal freely
- ⚠️ Family or friends comment that you're "too strict"
- ⚠️ You feel exhausted by the mental effort of perfect adherence

Signs you're being too flexible (more than 20 percent):

- ⚠️ Your weight loss has stalled for weeks
- ⚠️ You're gaining weight back
- ⚠️ "Flexible" meals are happening more than three or four times per week
- ⚠️ You're using flexibility as an excuse for emotional eating
- ⚠️ You don't track your adherence and can't honestly say what percentage you're following
- ⚠️ You feel out of control around food again

The goal: Find the balance where you're maintaining results while still enjoying life.

Quick-Win Challenge: Implementing Hack #7

Ready to add flexibility to your system? Here's how:

Step 1: Define Your 80 percent (Your Non-Negotiables)

Write down the habits you'll follow 80 percent of the time:

My non-negotiables:

- Intermittent fasting (16:8 minimum) most days
- Vegetables first when I eat
- Low-glycemic foods as primary fuel
- Meal prep on Sundays
- Seven-minute movement most mornings
- Real, whole foods (nothing processed)

What are yours? Be specific.

Step 2: Plan Your 20 percent (Your Flexibility Zones)

Decide when and how you'll be flexible.

Options:

- One weekend meal per week
- Special occasions only (birthdays, holidays, vacations)
- One planned treat per week
- Date nights with spouse/partner

What feels right for you? Write it down.

Step 3: Apply "Is This Special?"

This week, practice the question: "Is this special, or is it just available?"

When you're tempted by something off-plan, pause and ask:

- Is this a once-a-year experience, or can I have this anytime?
- Will I remember this meal in a month, or is it forgettable?
- Is this truly special to me, or am I eating it out of obligation/convenience?

Only say yes to truly special things.

Step 4: Practice Enjoying Without Guilt

Next time you have a flexible meal:

- Eat slowly
- Savor every bite
- Be fully present
- Enjoy the experience
- Do not allow guilt

Mental script: "I'm choosing to enjoy this. It's part of living a full, balanced life. Tomorrow, I'll return to my healthy habits."

Step 5: Return to 80 percent immediately.

This is where most people fail.

After your flexible meal, the very next meal should be completely on-plan:

- Vegetables first
- Low-glycemic

- Healthy fats and protein
- Intermittent fasting window maintained

No "I'll start Monday" mentality again. Start again at the very next meal.

Step 6: Track Your Balance Weekly

Every Sunday, reflect on the past week:

- How many meals followed your healthy habits?
- How many were flexible?
- What percentage does that represent?

Goal: 80 percent or higher adherence.

If you're below 80 percent, adjust. If you're above 95 percent, consider whether you're being too rigid.

Common Mistakes to Avoid

Mistake #1: Using 80/20 as an Excuse for Emotional Eating

The trap: "I'm feeling stressed, so I'm going to use my 20 percent and eat this entire pint of ice cream."

The truth: That's not flexibility—that's emotional eating disguised as flexibility.

The fix: Address the emotion (stress, sadness, boredom) directly. Save your 20 percent for planned, joyful experiences—not emotional Band-Aids. Chapter 10 provides detailed strategies for managing emotional eating.

Mistake #2: Flexible Meals Turning Into Flexible Days

The trap: "I had pizza for lunch, so the whole day is ruined. Might as well have ice cream tonight, too."

The truth: One meal doesn't ruin anything. But using it as an excuse to abandon all structure does.

The fix: Treat each meal independently. One flexible meal = one flexible meal. Period.

Mistake #3: Not Actually Tracking (and Being Closer to 50/50)

The trap: "I'm totally doing 80/20!" (But you're actually having six to eightflexible meals per week without realizing it.)

The truth: It's easy to underestimate how often you're being flexible, especially if you're not tracking.

The fix: Count your meals honestly every week. If you're consistently below 80 percent, your progress will stall.

Mistake #4: Choosing Low-Quality Treats

The trap: Wasting your 20 percent on gas station donuts or mediocre restaurant desserts.

The truth: Not all treats are created equal. Save your flexibility for truly special, high-quality indulgences.

The fix: Apply "Is this special?" ruthlessly. If it's not truly special, it's not worth your 20 percent.

Mistake #5: Feeling Guilty After Flexibility

The trap: Enjoying a planned treat, only to spend the next 24 hours feeling terrible about yourself.

The truth: Guilt destroys the benefit of flexibility and makes you more likely to spiral.

The fix: Practice enjoying without guilt. Remind yourself: "This is part of the plan. I'm living a balanced, sustainable life."

The Long Game: Why 80/20 Wins

Here's what I've learned after maintaining an 80-pound weight loss for over a decade:

- The people who succeed long-term aren't the most disciplined. They're the most flexible.
- The ultra-strict dieters? They lose weight fast. But then they burn out, binge, and gain it all back.
- The 80/20 practitioners? They lose weight steadily. And they keep it off forever.

The 80/20 Principle is sustainable. It's a lifestyle, not a diet. You win the long game not by being perfect, but by being consistent, flexible, and human.

What's Next?

You now have all 7 Hacks:

1. ☑ Eat Your Vegetables First
2. ☑ Make Low-Glycemic Swaps
3. ☑ Intermittent Fasting Made Easy
4. ☑ Turn Your Life Into a Fitness Routine
5. ☑ Embrace Healthy Fats and Unlock Ketosis
6. ☑ The Science Behind Meal Prep and Real Food
7. ☑ The 80/20 Flexibility Principle

These seven strategies, working together, create a complete system for insulin control, sustainable weight loss, and lasting metabolic health.

But knowing the hacks isn't enough.

In Chapter 10, we'll talk about maintenance—how to keep the weight off for life, how to handle plateaus, how to navigate the inevitable challenges, and how to truly shift your identity from "person who lost weight" to "healthy person who lives this way naturally."

Because losing weight is only half the battle. Keeping it off forever? That's where the real work begins.

CHAPTER 10

MAINTAINING YOUR RESULTS FOR LIFE

You did it.

You implemented the 7 Hacks. You lost the weight. You feel better than you have in years.

Your energy is up. Your clothes fit. People are noticing. You're proud of what you've accomplished.

But now comes the real question: *How do you keep it off?*

This is where most people fail. They reach their goal weight, celebrate, then slowly—sometimes quickly—slide back into old habits. Within months, sometimes weeks, the weight returns.

I know because I've watched it happen to friends, family members, and colleagues. They lose 30, 40, 50 pounds. They're thrilled. And then, six months later, it's all back.

Why does this happen?

Because they treated weight loss as a temporary project rather than a permanent lifestyle shift.

They thought, "Once I lose the weight, I can go back to normal."

But here's the truth: "Normal" is what made you overweight in the first place.

If you go back to eating the way you used to eat, you'll go back to looking the way you used to look.

Maintenance isn't about returning to your old life. It's about embracing your new one.

In this chapter, I'm going to show you exactly how to maintain your results—not for months, but for years.

This is the chapter I wish I'd had when I first lost the weight. It would have saved me from some painful lessons I learned the hard way.

Let's make sure you don't have to learn them the hard way, too.

The Maintenance Mindset Shift

The most significant difference between people who keep weight off and people who regain it isn't willpower or discipline.

It's a mindset.

Specifically, it's the shift from "I'm trying to lose weight" to "I'm a healthy person who lives this way."

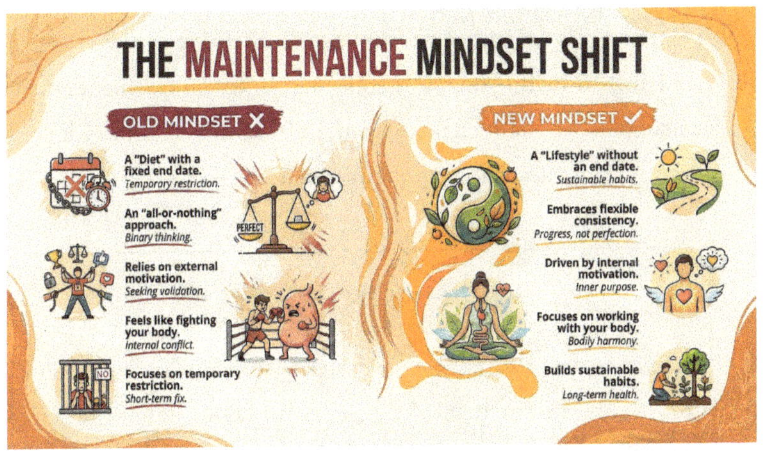

Two Very Different Identities

Identity #1: "I'm trying to lose weight."

This person thinks:

- "I *can't* eat that" (deprivation)
- "I *have to* work out" (obligation)
- "I *should* eat vegetables" (external pressure)
- "I'm *being good* today" (moralistic thinking)

This identity is temporary. It's something you're *doing*, not someone you *are*. And the moment you hit your goal weight, this identity loses its purpose. You've "succeeded," so you can stop now.

Identity #2: "I'm a healthy person."

This person thinks:

- "I *don't* eat that" (preference)
- "I *work out* every morning" (routine)
- "I *eat* vegetables first" (habit)
- "This is *how I live*" (identity)

This identity is permanent. It's not something you're doing temporarily—it's who you are. People who internalize this identity don't struggle with maintenance because they're not "maintaining"— they're just living according to their values.

📄 TRACK YOUR PROGRESS

Tracking creates awareness. I've designed The Fix Your Insulin Habit Scorecard to help you score your daily habits, build winning streaks, and maintain your results for life.

If you haven't already, download your free Habit Scorecard to track your journey over the next 8 weeks.

It's designed to help you build sustainable habits without overwhelm — one Hack at a time.

Get it free at:

FixYourInsulin.com/bonus

Scan with your phone's camera or visit the link above.

The Bridge: From "I Lost Weight" to "I Am a Healthy Person"

So how do you make this shift?

It happens through three practices:

Practice #1: Change Your Language

The words you use shape how you think about yourself.

Stop saying:

- "I'm *trying* to lose weight."
- "I'm *on* a diet."
- "I *can't* eat that."
- "I'm *being good* today."

Start saying:

- "I'm a healthy person."
- "This is how I eat."
- "I don't eat that"
- "I take care of my body."

Notice the difference? The first set of phrases implies effort, restriction, and temporality. The second set implies identity, preference, and permanence.

Your language creates your reality. Change how you talk about yourself, and you'll change how you see yourself.

Practice #2: Visualize Your Future Self

Close your eyes and imagine yourself five years from now.

There are two possible futures:

Future #1: You're back where you started. The weight returned. You feel defeated, frustrated, and stuck. You think, "I knew I couldn't keep it off."

Future #2: You're still healthy, energized, and fit. You've maintained your weight effortlessly. You think, "This is just who I am now."

The person in Future #2 isn't trying harder than the person in Future #1. They identify differently.

They don't see healthy eating as a chore—they see it as an expression of who they are.

Visualize that version of yourself. Then ask: What would *that* person do today? Would they skip their morning movement routine? Would they eat fast food for lunch? Would they stay up late binge-watching TV instead of getting restorative sleep?

No. Because that's not who they are.

Start acting as that future version of yourself today.

Practice #3: Embrace the Identity Through Action

Identity doesn't shift through thinking alone. It shifts through repeated action.

Every time you:

- Eat vegetables first

- Complete your morning Tabata
- Choose water over soda
- Meal prep on Sunday
- Fast until noon

You're casting a vote for the identity: "I am a healthy person."

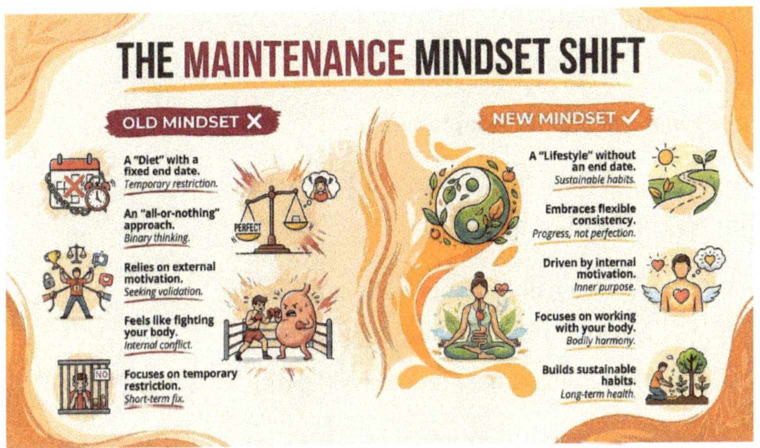

And the more votes you cast, the more solid that identity becomes.

Eventually, it's no longer something that takes effort to maintain. It's just who you are.

Breaking Through Plateaus

Even with perfect adherence, you will hit plateaus. Your weight will stall for weeks, sometimes months.

This is normal. This is expected. And it does NOT mean the system stopped working.

Why Plateaus Happen

Reason #1: Your Body Adapted

When you lose significant weight, your body requires fewer calories to function. A 200-pound body burns more calories at rest than a 160-pound body.

This doesn't mean your metabolism is "broken"—it's just adjusting to your smaller size.

Reason #2: Metabolic Adaptation

Your body is brilliant. When you lose weight, your body tries to prevent further loss by:

- Slightly reducing metabolic rate
- Increasing hunger hormones (ghrelin)
- Decreasing satiety hormones (leptin)

This is evolutionary survival programming. Your body thinks you're in a famine and is trying to protect you.

Reason #3: You're Losing Fat but Gaining Muscle

If you're doing resistance training (which you should be), you might be building muscle while losing fat. Muscle is denser than fat, so the scale might not move—but your body composition is improving.

Reason #4: Water Retention

Fat loss isn't linear. Sometimes your body temporarily holds onto water, masking fat loss on the scale.

Seven Strategies to Break Through Plateaus

When you hit a plateau that lasts three or more weeks, try the following strategies.

Strategy #1: Tighten Your Adherence

Be brutally honest: Are you truly following the hacks 80 percent of the time?

Often, plateaus happen because we've unconsciously drifted from 80/20 to 70/30 or 60/40.

Action steps:

- Track every meal for one week
- Count how many meals follow your healthy habits
- If you're below 80 percent, that's your answer

Strategy #2: Try Extended Fasting

If you're doing 16:8 intermittent fasting, try 18:6 or 20:4 for five to seven days.

Or try OMAD (One Meal A Day) two or three times per week.

Extended fasting gives your body a longer period of metabolic rest.

Strategy #3: Increase Movement Intensity

If you've been doing the same seven-minute Tabata for months, your body has adapted.

Options:

- Add a second movement session in the afternoon

- Increase Tabata intensity (go harder during work intervals)
- Add two resistance training sessions per week
- Take a 30-minute walk after dinner

More movement = more calories burned = plateau broken.

Strategy #4: Carb Cycling

If you've been eating very low-carb for months, try strategic carb refeeds:

Option A: One higher-carb day per week (100 to 150g carbs from sweet potato, quinoa, fruit)

Option B: Two moderate-carb days per week (75 to 100g carbs)

Carb refeeds can boost leptin, support thyroid function, and reset metabolic adaptation.

Strategy #5: Measure Differently

Sometimes the scale doesn't move, but your body is changing.

Track these instead:

- Body measurements (waist, hips, chest, arms)
- How your clothes fit
- Progress photos (front, side, back)
- Energy levels and how you feel

You might be losing inches even if the scale is stuck.

Strategy #6: Be Patient

Plateaus lasting two to four weeks are normal. Your body is adjusting.

Don't panic. Don't quit. Just stay consistent.

Often, plateaus break suddenly—you'll wake up one morning and suddenly be down two or three pounds.

Trust the process.

Strategy #7: Consider Timing

For women: Weight fluctuates significantly with menstrual cycles. You might retain water for seven to 10 days before your period, then drop several pounds after.

Track your cycle alongside your weight. You might discover your "plateau" is just hormonal water retention.

Navigating Life's Challenges

Maintenance isn't just about food and exercise. It's about handling the situations that tempt you to abandon your healthy habits.

Here's how to navigate the most common challenges.

Social Situations and Special Events

Dinner parties, weddings, holidays, and celebrations are minefields of temptation.

Before the event:

- Eat a small, protein-rich snack, so you're not starving

- Decide in advance what your boundaries are
- Remember: This is one meal, not a multi-day free-for-all

During the event:

- Start with vegetables if available
- Choose protein and fat options
- Limit alcohol to one or two drinks, if any
- Say no to foods that aren't "special" (use the "Is this special?" test from Chapter 9)
- Enjoy what you choose without guilt

After the event:

- Return to your healthy habits at the very next meal
- Don't weigh yourself the next day (you'll retain water)
- Move on mentally—no dwelling or guilt

Travel

Airports, hotels, and unfamiliar locations disrupt routines.

Airports:

- Pack protein snacks (nuts, jerky, cheese sticks)
- Skip the pastries, as they are usually not special
- Order salads or protein plates
- Stay hydrated

Hotels:

- Request a mini-fridge for your room
- Visit a local grocery store for healthy snacks
- Use hotel gyms or do bodyweight workouts in your room

- Maintain your fasting window

Restaurants:

- Skip the bread basket
- Ask for vegetables instead of fries/bread
- Order protein and vegetables, cooked simply
- Request dressings and sauces on the side
- Don't be shy about customizing orders

Holidays

Holidays always offer a challenge, but the end of the year is tough. Thanksgiving, Christmas, and New Year's are three food-centered celebrations that happen back-to-back.

Choose your indulgences:

- You don't have to eat everything at every meal
- Pick two or three truly special holiday foods and enjoy them
- Skip the mediocre stuff (store-bought cookies, generic candy)

Maintain structure:

- Keep your fasting window on non-celebration days
- Continue or even expand morning movement routines
- Eat vegetables first, even at holiday meals

Focus on connection, not food:

- Holidays are about people, not just eating
- Engage in activities beyond meals
- Volunteer, play games, take walks

Stressful Periods

Work deadlines, family crises, and financial stress—life happens, and stress eating calls.

Recognize emotional eating patterns:

- Ask: "Am I physically hungry, or am I feeling an emotion?"
- If it's emotion, food won't solve it

Stress management toolkit:

1. Ten-minute walk outside
2. Deep breathing (4-7-8 technique)
3. Call a friend
4. Journal your feelings
5. Take a hot shower
6. Go to bed early

Maintain non-negotiables:

- Even in chaos, protect sleep
- Even stressed, keep fasting windows
- Even if busy, do seven minutes of movement

Stress passes. Your healthy habits anchor you through it.

Regular Check-Ins: Your Early Warning System

The people who maintain weight loss long-term have early warning systems—they catch small gains before they become big problems.

Here's how to create yours.

Weekly Check-Ins

Every Sunday morning:

1. Weigh yourself (same day, same time, after using the bathroom, before eating)
2. Review the week: How many meals followed your healthy habits?
3. Plan the week: Meal prep, social events, potential challenges

Your "warning zone":

If your weight rises by 5 or more pounds outside your maintenance range, it's time to tighten up.

Don't wait until you've gained 20 pounds. Address it immediately.

Monthly Check-Ins

First Sunday of every month:

1. Take progress photos (front, side, back in the same clothes/ lighting.
2. Measure key areas (waist, hips, chest)
3. Reflect: What's working? What needs adjustment?
4. Celebrate wins: What are you proud of this month?

Monthly check-ins show trends that weekly weigh-ins might miss.

Quarterly Deep Dives

Every three months:

1. Get bloodwork (fasting insulin, A1C, lipid panel—if accessible)

2. Assess energy and mood: Are you thriving or just surviving?
3. Review your "why": Why did you start this journey? Are you honoring that?

Quarterly reviews keep you connected to the deeper purpose beyond the scale.

Your Maintenance Toolbox

Maintenance requires tools. Here are the ones I rely on most.

Tool #1: The 24-Hour Reset

When to use it: After a particularly indulgent meal or day

How it works:

The following 24 hours, you go strict:

- Extended fasting (20 or more hours if possible)
- First meal: vegetables only or a small salad with protein
- Second meal: vegetables first, then protein and fat, minimal carbs
- Extra movement (add a walk)

This resets insulin quickly and prevents one flexible day from becoming a flexible week.

Tool #2: The Weekly Meal Count

When to use it: When you suspect you're drifting from 80/20

How it works:

Count every meal for one week:

- Meals following healthy habits = _____
- Flexible meals = _____
- Percentage = _____

If you're below 80 percent, you know precisely where to tighten up.

Tool #3: The Morning Routine Anchor

When to use it: Always—this is your daily non-negotiable

How it works:

No matter what else happens, you do your seven-minute morning movement routine.

Why it matters: This small daily win builds momentum for healthy choices throughout the day.

Tool #4: The 80 percent Rule Reminder

When to use it: When you're tempted to overeat, even healthy foods

How it works:

Stop eating at 80 percent full. Push the plate away.

This prevents overeating and keeps portions in check—critical for maintenance.

Tool #5: The "Is This Special?" Question

When to use it: Every time you're tempted by something off-plan

How it works:

Ask yourself: "Is this special, or just available?"

If it's not truly special, it's not worth your 20 percent.

Tool #6: The Support System

When to use it: When you're struggling, tempted, or need accountability

How it works:

Identify two or three people who support your health goals:

- A spouse or partner
- A friend on a similar journey
- A family member who encourages you

Tell them when you're struggling. Ask for encouragement. Connection is medicine.

What to Do When You Slip Up

You will slip up. Everyone does.

You'll have a week where you abandon all structure. You'll go on vacation and gain seven pounds. You'll stress-eat your way through a family crisis.

This doesn't mean you've failed. It means you're human.

Here's exactly what to do when it happens.

Step 1: Acknowledge Without Judgment

Don't say: "I'm such a failure. I have no willpower. I knew I couldn't keep this up."

Do say: "I had a rough week. That's okay. I'm human. Now I'm getting back on track."

No shame. No guilt. Just acknowledgment and a decision to move forward.

Step 2: Identify the Trigger

Ask yourself: What caused this slip-up?

- Stress?
- Social pressure?
- Boredom?
- Lack of preparation?
- Emotional pain?

Understanding the trigger helps you prevent it next time.

Step 3: Return to Basics Immediately

Don't wait until Monday. Don't say "I'll start fresh next month."

Start at the very next meal.

Go back to the 7 Hacks.

Immediate action prevents a slip from becoming a slide.

Step 4: Use the 24-Hour Reset

After a particularly bad slip-up, employ the 24-Hour Reset tool explained above. This quickly brings insulin back under control.

Step 5: Forgive Yourself and Move On

The slip-up is in the past. You can't change it.

What you *can* change is what you do next.

Dwelling on guilt keeps you stuck. Forgiving yourself and taking action moves you forward.

You're not defined by one bad week. You're defined by how you respond.

The Long Game: Thinking in Years, Not Weeks

When I stopped thinking in weeks and started thinking in decades, everything changed.

Most people ask: "How do I get through this week without slipping up?"

I ask: "How do I want to feel when I'm 70 years old?"

My Vision for My Future Self

At 70, I want to be able to:

- Play with my grandchildren without getting winded
- Hike, travel, and stay active
- Be independent—not reliant on medications or caregivers

- Have energy and mental clarity
- Look back and think: "I took care of myself"

That vision guides every decision I make today.

When I'm tempted to skip my morning workout, I think: "Will skipping this help 70-year-old me?"

When I'm tempted to binge on junk food, I ask: "Is this honoring the future I want?"

The answer is always clear.

Your Long Game

Take a moment and envision your future self at 70, 80, or 90.

What do you want that person's life to look like?

- Vibrant and active, or frail and dependent?
- Energized and engaged, or exhausted and medicated?
- Proud of how you lived, or regretful about neglect?

The choices you make today create that future.

Eat every vegetable first. Every morning, you move your body. Every time you choose real food over processed junk.

You're not just maintaining weight. You're building the rest of your life.

Maintenance Is Not a Burden—It's a Gift

Most people see maintenance as:

- A chore

- Something to endure
- A constant battle

I see it as a gift.

The gift of:

- Waking up with energy
- Fitting into clothes I love
- Playing actively with my kids
- Feeling confident in my body
- Knowing I'm taking care of myself
- Living fully without being limited by weight

Maintenance isn't restricting my life. It's enabling my life.

Every healthy choice I make isn't a sacrifice—it's an investment in more years of vitality, energy, and joy.

When you see it this way, maintenance stops feeling like deprivation and becomes a form of self-respect.

You've Got This

Maintaining weight loss for life isn't about perfection.

It's about:

- Showing up consistently
- Catching small slips before they become big ones
- Having tools ready for challenges
- Thinking long-term, not just week-to-week
- Identifying as a healthy person, not someone "trying" to be healthy

You've already done the hard part—you lost the weight.

Now you need to protect what you've built.

And with the identity shift, the tools, and the strategies in this chapter, you absolutely can.

In Chapter 11, we'll explore what life looks like beyond weight loss—the more profound transformations in energy, confidence, relationships, and purpose that happen when you sustain this lifestyle long-term.

Because this journey isn't just about losing weight.

It's about reclaiming your life.

Let's talk about what that looks like.

CHAPTER 11

YOUR NEW LIFE: BEYOND WEIGHT LOSS

When I started this journey at 280 pounds, I thought weight loss was the goal.

Lose the weight. Fit into smaller clothes. Look better. Feel less embarrassed. Maybe improve my health markers enough to get off medications.

That's what I thought I was signing up for.

But what I discovered was something far more profound: Weight loss wasn't the destination—it was the doorway to an entirely new life.

Yes, the number on the scale changed, but everything else changed too—in ways I never expected.

My energy transformed. My relationships deepened. My career flourished. My confidence soared. My entire relationship with my body, food, and health shifted from fear and restriction to trust and abundance. I became more radiant, my self-esteem grew, and my confidence solidified. I started to feel almost invincible—not in an arrogant way, but in a deeply grounded sense of capability and strength. That magical feeling of accomplishment—of proving to myself that I could transform my life—was intoxicating.

Losing 80 pounds changed my body. But the journey changed my life.

And now, as you implement these 7 Hacks and experience your own transformation, you're discovering the same truth: This isn't just about weight loss. It's about reclaiming your vitality, your confidence, and your future.

Welcome to Chapter 11: Your New Life: Beyond Weight Loss.

This is where we explore what happens when you stick with this journey long enough for the real magic to unfold. This is about the ripple effects that extend far beyond the scale—into your health, energy, relationships, career, and sense of purpose.

The Health Benefits You'll Experience

Let's start with the most obvious—but still remarkable—transformation: your health.

When you follow the 7 Hacks in this book, you're not just losing weight; you're addressing the root cause of metabolic dysfunction: insulin resistance.

And when you fix insulin, everything else starts to heal.

Blood Sugar and Insulin Sensitivity

What happens:

- Your fasting insulin levels drop
- Your blood sugar stabilizes
- Your A1C (a measure of long-term blood sugar control) improves
- Your risk of Type 2 diabetes decreases significantly

What you notice:

- Fewer afternoon energy crashes
- Fewer „hangry" meltdowns
- More steady, reliable energy throughout the day
- Mental clarity that feels almost superhuman

Within months of implementing these hacks, my fasting insulin went from dangerously high to completely normal. My doctor was shocked. I felt like I'd been given a new operating system—everything just worked better.

Cardiovascular Health

What happens:

- Your blood pressure normalizes
- Your triglycerides drop
- Your HDL (good cholesterol) increases
- Your LDL particle size improves (small, dense particles become large, fluffy ones)
- Inflammation markers like C-reactive protein decline

What you notice:

- Fewer or no heart palpitations
- Better stamina and endurance
- Feeling lighter and less congested
- Climbing stairs without getting winded

My blood pressure went from pre-hypertensive to optimal. My cardiologist said, "Whatever you're doing, keep doing it." The transformation in my cardiovascular health gave me hope for a long, active life.

Important note: If you have existing cardiovascular conditions or take heart medications, please work closely with your healthcare provider as you implement these changes. Your doctor may need to adjust medications as your health improves.

Inflammation and Pain Reduction

Excess weight, especially around the midsection, produces inflammatory chemicals. When you lose that weight—primarily through insulin control—inflammation decreases significantly.

What happens:

- Joint pain decreases
- Chronic inflammation subsides
- Autoimmune symptoms may improve
- Recovery from exercise speeds up

What you notice:

- Your joints stop hurting
- Back pain diminishes or disappears

- You wake up feeling refreshed, not stiff and achy
- Old injuries stop nagging you

I used to wake up every morning with lower back pain. I accepted it as a sign of "just getting older." Within two months of this journey, it was gone. Completely. I realized it wasn't age—it was inflammation and excess weight stressing my body.

Hormonal Balance

When insulin is high, it disrupts other hormones—thyroid, sex hormones, and stress hormones. Fix insulin, and the entire hormonal orchestra starts playing in harmony.

What happens:

- Testosterone levels normalize for men
- Estrogen and progesterone balance for women
- Thyroid function improves
- Cortisol (stress hormone) regulates
- Growth hormone increases

What you notice:

- Better sleep quality
- Improved libido
- More stable mood
- Increased muscle mass
- Better stress resilience

My energy, mood, and vitality improved so dramatically that my wife joked, "I feel like I got my husband back." Hormones matter more than most people realize.

Longevity and Disease Prevention

The habits you're building don't just help you lose weight—they're some of the most powerful longevity interventions known to science.

What the research suggests:

- Intermittent fasting activates autophagy (cellular cleanup)
- Low-glycemic eating reduces oxidative stress
- Healthy fats support brain health and reduce dementia risk
- Movement and strength training preserve muscle and bone density
- Insulin control reduces cancer risk

What this means:

- You're not just living longer—you're living better
- You're compressing morbidity (staying healthy until the very end, rather than declining for decades)
- You're reducing your risk of Alzheimer's, cancer, heart disease, and stroke
- You're giving yourself the best chance at a vibrant, independent old age

I used to think about health in terms of "not being sick." Now I think about it in terms of thriving at 70, 80, 90, or older. I want to be the grandparent who plays with grandkids, travels the world, and lives fully until the very end.

The Energy Revolution

One of the most dramatic—and immediate—benefits you'll experience is energy.

Not the jittery, caffeine-fueled, crash-later energy, but steady, sustained, powerful energy that carries you through the day with clarity and strength.

Why Your Energy Transforms

1. Stable blood sugar = stable energy

When you eat low-glycemic foods and control insulin, your blood sugar doesn't spike and crash. You're running on premium fuel, not sugar-coated roller coasters.

2. Fat-burning efficiency

When your body is adapted to burning fat (through ketosis or low-carb eating), you have access to nearly unlimited energy. Fat stores are abundant. Glucose stores are limited. Fat = endurance.

3. Reduced inflammation

Inflammation is exhausting. It's your body in constant repair mode. When inflammation drops, energy soars.

4. Better sleep

Weight loss, especially around the neck and midsection, reduces sleep apnea and improves sleep quality. Better sleep = better energy.

5. Hormonal optimization

Balanced hormones mean your body produces and utilizes energy more efficiently.

I used to need two large coffees to get through the morning, and I'd still be yawning by 2 p.m. Now? I have one black coffee in the morning because I enjoy it, not because I need it. My energy is consistent from 6 a.m. to 10 p.m. It's like upgrading from a flip phone to a smartphone—everything works better.

The Mental Clarity Breakthrough

This one surprised me the most.

I expected weight loss. I hoped for better health. But I didn't anticipate the dramatic improvement in mental clarity, focus, and cognitive function.

***Why Your Brain Gets Sharper**

1. Ketones are brain fuel

When you're in ketosis or low-carb, your liver produces ketones—and your brain loves them. Many people report feeling sharper, more focused, and more creative in ketosis.

2. Reduced brain fog from blood sugar swings

High blood sugar followed by crashes creates cognitive dysfunction. Stable blood sugar = stable cognition.

3. Reduced inflammation

Inflammation affects the brain as much as the body. Lower inflammation = better mood, memory, and mental performance.

4. Better sleep

Deep, restorative sleep is when your brain consolidates memories and clears out metabolic waste. Better sleep = better brain function.

5. Increased Brain-Derived Neurotrophic Factor (BDNF)

Fasting and exercise increase BDNF, a protein that supports brain health, neuroplasticity, and mood regulation.

Within a month of starting intermittent fasting and a low-carb diet, I noticed I could focus for three to four hours straight without distractions. My creativity exploded. I started writing again—something I hadn't done in years because my mind felt too foggy. People at work commented on how sharp I'd become in meetings.

This isn't just anecdotal—there's real science behind it. Your brain is thriving.

The Confidence Transformation

Weight loss changes how you look, but it also changes how you feel about yourself—and how you show up in the world.

Physical Confidence

What happens:

- You move more freely and comfortably

- You're not self-conscious about your appearance
- You catch your reflection and think, "Hey, I look good!"

The ripple effects:

- You try new activities (hiking, dancing, sports)
- You're more willing to be in photos
- You engage more in social situations
- You carry yourself differently—your posture improves, and you have the confidence to take up space

I avoided photos for years. I'd delete pictures where I looked too heavy. Now? I take photos with my kids without hesitation. I'm present in memories instead of hiding from the camera.

Internal Confidence

The more profound shift is in internal confidence—the beliefs that you can set a goal and achieve it, that you're capable of change, and that you're in control of your life.

What happens:

- You prove to yourself: "I said I'd do this, and I did."
- You realize: "If I can do this, what else can I do?"
- You trust yourself more
- You stop making excuses in other areas of life

The ripple effects:

- You tackle other challenges (career, relationships, finances)
- You set bigger goals

- You inspire others
- You become the person people come to for advice

Losing 80 pounds taught me that I'm capable of complicated things. That lesson transferred everywhere. I asked for a promotion at work—and got it. I started projects I'd been putting off for years. I became more assertive in relationships. The confidence from weight loss became confidence in life.

The Relationship Ripple Effect

Your transformation doesn't happen in isolation. It affects everyone around you—especially the people closest to you.

Romantic Relationships

What improves:

- Physical intimacy: Increased energy, libido, and confidence
- Emotional connection: You're happier, less irritable, more present
- Shared activities: You can do more together—hiking, traveling, playing with kids
- Mutual respect: Your partner appreciates your commitment and discipline

Potential challenges:

- Your partner may feel threatened or insecure
- You may outgrow the relationship dynamic
- They may resist your changes or try to sabotage (subconsciously)

How to navigate:

- Communicate openly about your goals and why they matter
- Invite your partner to join you (but don't force it)
- Reassure them that your transformation strengthens the relationship
- Seek couples support if needed

My wife was my biggest supporter. She naturally started adopting some of my habits—not because I pushed, but because she saw the results. We became an even better team. Our relationship deepened because I was healthier, happier, and more present.

Family Dynamics

What improves:

- Your kids see you modeling healthy habits naturally
- Family meals become teaching moments about nutrition and food choices
- You're more active and energetic with your children—playing, hiking, being present
- You're breaking generational patterns of poor health that may have affected your family for decades

Potential challenges:

- Children may resist changes to familiar foods or meal routines
- Family members might feel judged by your new habits
- Meal preparation becomes more complex when cooking different foods for different family members

- Your partner or kids may not support or understand your journey, especially initially

How to navigate:

- Lead by example rather than lecturing—let them see your results
- Involve kids in meal prep and grocery shopping to build their interest
- Make gradual changes to family meals rather than overnight overhauls
- Communicate openly with your partner about why this matters to you and your family's future
- Be flexible—use the 80/20 rule for family celebrations and special occasions
- Focus on adding healthy options rather than restricting what others eat

My kids started asking questions: "Why do you eat vegetables first?" "Why don't we have soda?" Instead of lecturing, I just modeled the behavior and piqued their curiosity. Now they naturally make better choices. I'm breaking a cycle of poor health that ran in my family for generations.

Friendships and Social Circles

What shifts:

- Some friends will be inspired and supportive
- Others may feel judged or uncomfortable

- You might naturally gravitate toward people with similar health values
- You may outgrow friendships based on unhealthy habits

How to navigate:

- Don't preach or judge
- Lead by example
- Be flexible in social situations (80/20 principle)
- Find new communities aligned with your values

Some friendships faded—especially those centered on drinking and poor eating. But new friendships were formed with people who valued health, growth, and intentional living. The quality of my social life improved dramatically.

The Career and Productivity Boost

This is another unexpected benefit: your professional life improves.

Why This Happens

1. More energy and stamina

You can work longer, think more clearly, and handle stress better.

2. Improved focus and productivity

Mental clarity translates to better decision-making and problem-solving.

3. Greater confidence

You're more willing to speak up, take on challenges, and pursue opportunities.

4. Better presence and charisma

People notice when you're energized, confident, and engaged.

5. Discipline transfers

The discipline you built for losing weight shows up in your work ethic.

Within six months of my transformation, I was promoted. My boss said, "You've become a different person—more confident, more reliable, more leadership-oriented." I'm convinced my health transformation directly contributed to my career success.

The Deeper Purpose That Emerges

Once you reclaim your health, you start asking bigger questions.

Before, you were trying to survive. You wanted to lose some weight, feel less terrible, and get through the day.

After you reclaim your health, you begin thriving. And you start wondering: "What am I here to do? What's my purpose? How can I contribute?"

This happens because when you're unhealthy, all your energy goes to basic survival—managing pain, fatigue, illness, and self-consciousness. You're in reactive mode. But when you're healthy, you have surplus energy and mental bandwidth to think beyond yourself. You shift from survival to contribution.

What This Looks Like

- You start mentoring others who want to lose weight
- You become an example in your community
- You pursue passions you'd abandoned
- You take risks you wouldn't have before
- You ask: "What legacy do I want to leave?"

After losing 80 pounds and maintaining it for years, people started asking me for advice. At first, I'd share casually. But over time, I realized this knowledge can help so many people. That's why I wrote this book. My transformation gave me purpose beyond myself—to help others transform, too.

Living Fully: The Ultimate Benefit

At the end of the day, this journey is about one thing: living fully.

Not just existing. Not just surviving. But thriving.

Living fully means:

- Playing with your kids or grandkids without getting winded
- Traveling without worrying about airplane seatbelts or walking long distances
- Trying new activities without fear or embarrassment
- Feeling confident in your own skin
- Having the energy to pursue your dreams
- Being present in every moment

My defining moment was six months into my journey, when my daughter asked if I'd go on a hike with her. The old me would've made excuses. The new me said yes right away. We hiked five miles together, talking and laughing the whole way. At the top of the mountain, looking out over the valley, I realized: This is what I've been missing. This is why it matters.

Not the number on the scale. Not fitting into more petite jeans, but being able to participate in life fully.

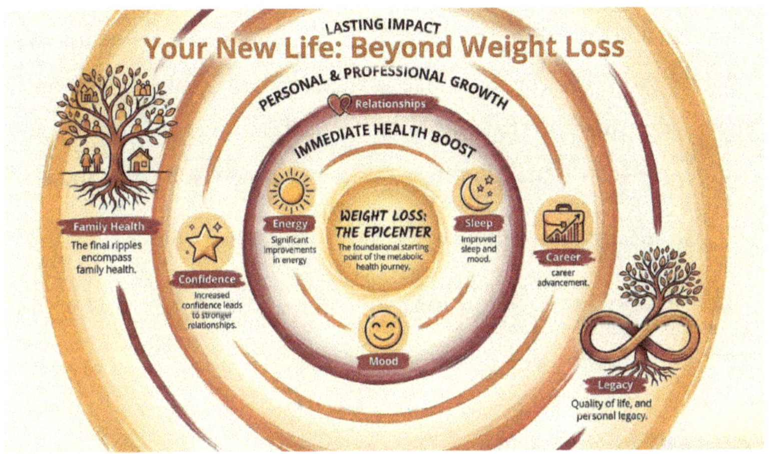

The Journey Never Ends—And That's Beautiful

This isn't a finish line. It's a way of life.

There's no point where you "arrive" and stop. Health is something you practice daily, for the rest of your life.

But that's not a burden—it's a gift.

Because every day, you get to choose: Will I honor my body today? Will I nourish it, move it, rest it, care for it?

And every time you choose yes, you're reinforcing the identity: "I am a healthy person."

The Habits Become Who You Are

At first, eating vegetables first feels like a strategy. Over time, it becomes automatic.

At first, intermittent fasting requires discipline. Over time, you don't even think about it. In fact, one of my greatest privileges nowadays is experiencing real hunger again. I've come to appreciate that feeling—it makes me feel alive and grateful for the opportunity to nourish my body with healthy food that I can savor, bite by bite. That's how my relationship with food has transformed. Hunger isn't the enemy anymore—it's a signal that my body is working exactly as it should.

At first, meal prep feels like work. Over time, it becomes meditative.

The 7 Hacks stop being things you "do" and start being who you "are."

A Final Reflection

When I stood on that scale at 280 pounds, hearing my doctor's warning about heart disease and diabetes, I felt hopeless.

I thought: "This is it. This is who I am. I'm just a fat guy who's going to be sick and die young."

But I was wrong.

I wasn't broken. I wasn't doomed. I didn't have the correct information. But I got that information and changed my life.

And now, *you* have that information, too.

You have the 7 Hacks that can transform your body, your health, and your life.

You have the knowledge that it's not about willpower—it's about insulin.

You have the tools to lose weight without hunger, without calorie counting, without feeling deprived.

What you do with this information is up to you.

You can close this book, go back to your old habits, and hope things change on their own.

Or you can take action. Start with Hack #1 tomorrow. Eat your vegetables first. Then add Hack #2 next week. Implement hack by hack. Build momentum. Trust the process.

Your transformation is waiting.

Not someday. Not when conditions are perfect. Not when you have more time or willpower.

Now.

FINAL WORD

You made it.

The fact that you're here, reading these final words, tells me something about you. You're not someone who gives up. You're not someone who settles for less than what you deserve. You're ready to change—truly change—and reclaim the health, energy, and life you were meant to live.

And I'm honored to have been part of your journey.

This Is Just the Beginning

Closing this book doesn't mean the journey ends. In fact, your journey is just beginning.

Tomorrow morning, you'll wake up with a choice: Will I start implementing these hacks, or will I go back to old patterns?

I hope—deeply—that you choose to start.

You don't need to overhaul your entire life overnight. You need to take the first step. And then the next. And then the next.

Small, consistent actions compound into extraordinary results.

Stay Curious, Keep Learning

This book gave you the foundation, but health is a lifelong practice, and there's always more to learn.

Stay curious. Read more books. Listen to podcasts. Follow researchers and practitioners who align with evidence-based approaches to metabolic health.

Keep experimenting with what works for *your* body. Not every strategy will resonate with everyone. Some people thrive in deep ketosis. Others do better with moderate low-carb. Some love OMAD. Others prefer 16:8.

Your body is your laboratory. Pay attention. Track what makes you feel amazing. Adjust what doesn't serve you.

Health is personal. There's no one-size-fits-all.

But the principles in this book—insulin control, real food, metabolic rest, movement, flexibility—these are universal. Build on this foundation and make it your own.

My Promise to You

I can't promise you'll lose 80 pounds as I did. Everyone's journey is different.

But I can promise this:

If you implement these 7 Hacks consistently, your life will change.

Your energy will improve. Your cravings will diminish. Your health markers will get better. Your confidence will grow.

You'll feel more alive than you have in years.

And that feeling—that vibrant, energized, capable feeling—will motivate you to keep going.

The results will fuel the commitment. The commitment will deepen the results.

It's a beautiful upward spiral, and you're about to experience it.

One Final Encouragement

Fourteen years ago, I stood on a scale at 280 pounds, terrified and hopeless.

I didn't believe I could change. I thought I was destined to be overweight and unhealthy for the rest of my life.

But I was wrong.

And if you're feeling that same hopelessness right now, you're wrong too.

You *can* do this.

Your body is incredibly resilient. It wants to heal. It wants to thrive. You need to give it the right inputs—the right food, the right timing, the proper movement, the right rest.

Your transformation is not only possible—it's inevitable, as long as you stay consistent.

So take a deep breath. Commit. Start tomorrow.

Your new life is waiting.

WHAT'S NEXT?

Thank you for reading Fix Your Insulin.

I hope the 7 Hacks serve you as well as they've served me.

Your journey doesn't end here.

I'm building something new — an AI-powered tool to give you personalized guidance based on the principles in this book.

Think of it as having me in your pocket, ready to answer your questions about food choices, meal timing, and troubleshooting plateaus.

If you'd like to be first to know when it launches (and get exclusive early access), visit:

AskKarlJacob.com

I'd love to hear how the 7 Hacks are working for you.

Stay healthy,

Karl

REFERENCES AND SCIENTIFIC SUPPORT

This book is grounded in peer-reviewed research, clinical studies, and evidence-based science. Below are key references supporting the 7 Hacks and core concepts presented throughout the book.

INSULIN RESISTANCE AND METABOLIC HEALTH

1. Reaven, G. M. (1988). "Banting lecture 1988. Role of insulin resistance in human disease." *Diabetes*, 37(12), 1595-1607.
    - Foundational research on insulin resistance and metabolic syndrome
2. Ludwig, D. S., & Ebbeling, C. B. (2018). "The Carbohydrate-Insulin Model of Obesity: Beyond 'Calories In, Calories Out.'" *JAMA Internal Medicine*, 178(8), 1098-1103.
    - Challenges the calories-in/calories-out model; emphasizes insulin's role in obesity
3. Taubes, G. (2016). *The Case Against Sugar*. New York: Alfred A. Knopf.
    - Comprehensive examination of sugar's role in metabolic disease
4. Fung, J., & Moore, J. (2016). *The Obesity Code: Unlocking the Secrets of Weight Loss*. Vancouver: Greystone Books.
    - Clinical perspective on insulin resistance and weight loss

HACK #1: FOOD ORDER (VEGETABLES FIRST)

1. Imai, S., et al. (2011). "A simple meal plan of 'eating vegetables before carbohydrate' was more effective for achieving glycemic control than an exchange-based meal plan in Japanese patients with type 2 diabetes." *Asia Pacific Journal of Clinical Nutrition*, 20(2), 161-168.

   • Demonstrates the vegetables-before-carbs approach for glycemic control

2. Imai, S., et al. (2014). "Eating vegetables before carbohydrates improves postprandial glucose excursions." *European Journal of Clinical Nutrition*, 68(5), 582-588.

   • Study 2 cited in Chapter 3—Japanese research showing that vegetables and protein before rice significantly lowers post-meal blood sugar in Type 2 diabetes patients

3. Shukla, A. P., et al. (2015). "Food Order Has a Significant Impact on Postprandial Glucose and Insulin Levels." *Diabetes Care*, 38(7), e98-e99.

   • Study 1 cited in Chapter 3—Weill Cornell Medical College research showing a 73 percent reduction in glucose spikes and 48 percent reduction in insulin spikes when eating vegetables before carbohydrates

4. Shukla, A. P., et al. (2017). "Carbohydrate-last meal pattern lowers postprandial glucose and insulin excursions in type 2 diabetes." *BMJ Open Diabetes Research & Care*, 5(1), e000440.

   • Further evidence that food order matters for blood sugar control

5. Tricò, D., et al. (2016). "Manipulating the sequence of food ingestion improves glycemic control in type 2 diabetic patients under free-living conditions." *Nutrition & Diabetes*, 6(8), e226.

   • Real-world application of food order strategy

GASTRIC EMPTYING AND MACRONUTRIENT EFFECTS

1. Gentilcore, D., et al. (2006). "Effects of fat, protein, and carbohydrate and protein load on blood glucose and plasma GLP-1 and ghrelin." *American Journal of Clinical Nutrition*, 84(1), 146-152.

   • Study 3 concept—shows protein and fat slow gastric emptying and reduces glucose response

2. Ma, J., et al. (2009). "Effects of a protein preload on gastric emptying, glycemia, and gut hormones after a carbohydrate meal in diet-controlled type 2 diabetes." *Diabetes Care*, 32(9), 1600-1602.

   • Protein consumed before carbohydrates significantly reduces postprandial glucose

3. Kuwata, H., et al. (2016). "Meal sequence and glucose excursion, gastric emptying and incretin secretion in type 2 diabetes: a randomised, controlled crossover, exploratory trial." *Diabetologia*, 59(3), 453-461.

   • Demonstrates that eating protein/vegetables before carbohydrates slows gastric emptying and improves glucose control

HACK #2: LOW-GLYCEMIC SWAPS

1. Jenkins, D. J., et al. (1981). "Glycemic index of foods: a physiological basis for carbohydrate exchange." *American Journal of Clinical Nutrition,* 34(3), 362-366.
    * Original glycemic index research
2. Ludwig, D. S. (2002). "The glycemic index: physiological mechanisms relating to obesity, diabetes, and cardiovascular disease." *JAMA,* 287(18), 2414-2423.
    * Links glycemic index to obesity and metabolic disease
3. Brand-Miller, J., et al. (2003). *The New Glucose Revolution: The Authoritative Guide to the Glycemic Index.* New York: Marlowe & Company.
    * Comprehensive guide to glycemic index
4. Thomas, D. E., et al. (2007). "Low glycaemic index, or low glycaemic load, diets for diabetes mellitus." *Cochrane Database of Systematic Reviews,* 3, CD006296.
    * Meta-analysis showing benefits of low-glycemic eating for diabetes management

HACK #3: INTERMITTENT FASTING

1. Mattson, M. P., et al. (2017). "Impact of intermittent fasting on health and disease processes." *Ageing Research Reviews,* 39, 46-58.
    * Comprehensive review of intermittent fasting benefits
2. Anton, S. D., et al. (2018). "Flipping the Metabolic Switch: Understanding and Applying the Health Benefits of Fasting." *Obesity,* 26(2), 254-268.
    * Explains metabolic switching from glucose to ketones during fasting

3. de Cabo, R., & Mattson, M. P. (2019). "Effects of Intermittent Fasting on Health, Aging, and Disease." *New England Journal of Medicine*, 381(26), 2541-2551.

   • Clinical review of intermittent fasting for health and longevity

4. Sutton, E. F., et al. (2018). "Early Time-Restricted Feeding Improves Insulin Sensitivity, Blood Pressure, and Oxidative Stress Even without Weight Loss in Men with Prediabetes." *Cell Metabolism*, 27(6), 1212-1221.e3.

   • Shows intermittent fasting improves metabolic health independent of weight loss

5. Tinsley, G. M., & La Bounty, P. M. (2015). "Effects of intermittent fasting on body composition and clinical health markers in humans." *Nutrition Reviews*, 73(10), 661-674.

   • Review of intermittent fasting effects on body composition

AUTOPHAGY AND CELLULAR CLEANUP

1. Levine, B., & Kroemer, G. (2008). "Autophagy in the pathogenesis of disease." *Cell*, 132(1), 27-42.

   • Foundational research on autophagy and disease prevention

2. Alirezaei, M., et al. (2010). "Short-term fasting induces profound neuronal autophagy." *Autophagy*, 6(6), 702-710.

   • Shows fasting triggers autophagy in the brain

3. Longo, V. D., & Mattson, M. P. (2014). "Fasting: molecular mechanisms and clinical applications." *Cell Metabolism*, 19(2), 181-192.

   • Reviews fasting-induced autophagy and health benefits

HACK #4: MOVEMENT AND METABOLIC HEALTH

1. Borghouts, L. B., & Keizer, H. A. (2000). "Exercise and insulin sensitivity: a review." *International Journal of Sports Medicine*, 21(1), 1-12.

   • Reviews how exercise improves insulin sensitivity

2. Colberg, S. R., et al. (2010). "Exercise and type 2 diabetes: the American College of Sports Medicine and the American Diabetes Association: joint position statement." *Diabetes Care*, 33(12), e147-e167.

   • Evidence-based guidelines on exercise for diabetes

3. Reynolds, A. N., et al. (2016). "Advice to walk after meals is more effective for lowering postprandial glycaemia in type 2 diabetes mellitus than advice that does not specify timing: a randomised crossover study." *Diabetologia*, 59(12), 2572-2578.

   • Post-meal walking significantly reduces blood sugar spikes

4. Crum, A. J., & Langer, E. J. (2007). "Mind-set matters: exercise and the placebo effect." *Psychological Science*, 18(2), 165-171.

   • Hotel workers' study showing daily activity improves health markers

5. Gibala, M. J., et al. (2012). "Physiological adaptations to low-volume, high-intensity interval training in health and disease." *Journal of Physiology*, 590(5), 1077-1084.

   • Evidence for high-intensity interval training (HIIT/ Tabata)

HACK #5: HEALTHY FATS AND KETOSIS

1. Volek, J. S., & Phinney, S. D. (2011). *The Art and Science of Low-Carbohydrate Living.* Miami: Beyond Obesity LLC.

    • Comprehensive guide to ketogenic diets and fat metabolism

2. Paoli, A., et al. (2013). "Beyond weight loss: a review of the therapeutic uses of very-low-carbohydrate (ketogenic) diets." *European Journal of Clinical Nutrition*, 67(8), 789-796.

    • Reviews therapeutic benefits of ketogenic diets beyond weight loss

3. Yancy, W. S., et al. (2004). "A low-carbohydrate, ketogenic diet versus a low-fat diet to treat obesity and hyperlipidemia: a randomized, controlled trial." *Annals of Internal Medicine*, 140(10), 769-777.

    • Clinical trial showing ketogenic diet outperforms low-fat diet

4. Forsythe, C. E., et al. (2008). "Comparison of low-fat and low-carbohydrate diets on circulating fatty acid composition and markers of inflammation." *Lipids*, 43(1), 65-77.

    • Low-carb diet reduces inflammation more than a low-fat diet

5. Newman, J. C., & Verdin, E. (2017). "β-Hydroxybutyrate: A Signaling Metabolite." *Annual Review of Nutrition*, 37, 51-76.

    • Explains how ketones benefit the brain and body

6. Siri-Tarino, P. W., et al. (2010). "Meta-analysis of prospective cohort studies evaluating the association of saturated fat with cardiovascular disease." American Journal of Clinical Nutrition, 91(3), 535-546.

    • No significant association between saturated fat and heart disease

7. Mozaffarian, D., et al. (2010). "Effects on coronary heart disease of increasing polyunsaturated fat in place of saturated fat: a systematic review and meta-analysis of randomized controlled trials." *PLoS Medicine*, 7(3), e1000252.

    • Examines effects of different dietary fats

8. DiNicolantonio, J. J., & O'Keefe, J. H. (2018). "Effects of dietary fats on blood lipids: a review of direct comparison trials." *Open Heart*, 5(2), e000871.

    • Reviews how different fats affect cholesterol

HACK #6: The Science Behind Meal Prep and Real Food

1. Mozaffarian, D., et al. (2011). "Changes in diet and lifestyle and long-term weight gain in women and men." *New England Journal of Medicine*, 364(25), 2392-2404.

    • Links processed foods to weight gain; whole foods to weight maintenance

2. Monteiro, C. A., et al. (2019). "Ultra-processed foods, diet quality, and health using the NOVA classification system." *Rome*: FAO.

    • Classification system for processed foods and health impacts

3. Hall, K. D., et al. (2019). "Ultra-Processed Diets Cause Excess Calorie Intake and Weight Gain: An Inpatient Randomized Controlled Trial of Ad Libitum Food Intake." *Cell Metabolism*, 30(1), 67-77.e3.

    • Ultra-processed foods cause overeating compared to whole foods

4. Wolfson, J. A., & Bleich, S. N. (2015). "Is cooking at home associated with better diet quality or weight-loss intention?" *Public Health Nutrition*, 18(8), 1397-1406.

    - Home cooking is associated with better diet quality

HACK #7: 80/20 FLEXIBILITY AND SUSTAINABILITY

1. Stewart, T. M., et al. (2002). "Rigid vs. flexible dieting: association with eating disorder symptoms in nonobese women." *Appetite*, 38(1), 39-44.

    - Flexible dieting is associated with better psychological outcomes

2. Smith, C. F., et al. (1999). "Flexible vs. Rigid dieting strategies: relationship with adverse behavioral outcomes." *Appetite*, 32(3), 295-305.

    - Rigid dieting linked to binge eating and poor outcomes

3. Westenhoefer, J., et al. (2013). "Behavioural correlates of successful weight loss over 3 y. Results from the Lean Habits Study." *International Journal of Obesity*, 37(8), 1009-1015.

    - Flexible control predicts long-term weight maintenance

WEIGHT LOSS MAINTENANCE

1. Wing, R. R., & Phelan, S. (2005). "Long-term weight loss maintenance." *American Journal of Clinical Nutrition*, 82(1), 222S-225S.

    - Research from the National Weight Control Registry on successful maintainers

2. Thomas, J. G., et al. (2014). "Weight-loss maintenance for 10 years in the National Weight Control Registry." *American Journal of Preventive Medicine, 46(1), 17-23.*

   • Long-term maintenance strategies from successful individuals

MEAL TIMING AND CIRCADIAN RHYTHM

1. Garaulet, M., & Gómez-Abellán, P. (2014). "Timing of food intake and obesity: a novel association." *Physiology & Behavior*, 134, 44-50.

   • Meal timing affects weight and metabolism

2. Jakubowicz, D., et al. (2013). "High caloric intake at breakfast vs. dinner differentially influences weight loss of overweight and obese women." *Obesity*, 21(12), 2504-2512.

   • Eating earlier in the day is more effective for weight loss

3. Gill, S., & Panda, S. (2015). "A smartphone app reveals erratic diurnal eating patterns in humans that can be modulated for health benefits." *Cell Metabolism*, 22(5), 789-798.

   • Time-restricted eating improves health markers

SLEEP, STRESS, AND WEIGHT

1. Taheri, S., et al. (2004). "Short sleep duration is associated with reduced leptin, elevated ghrelin, and increased body mass index." *PLoS Medicine*, 1(3), e62.

   • Sleep deprivation affects hunger hormones

2. Spiegel, K., et al. (2004). "Brief communication: Sleep curtailment in healthy young men is associated with

decreased leptin levels, elevated ghrelin levels, and increased hunger and appetite." *Annals of Internal Medicine*, 141(11), 846-850.

- Poor sleep increases appetite

3. Epel, E. S., et al. (2000). "Stress and body shape: stress-induced cortisol secretion is consistently greater among women with central fat." *Psychosomatic Medicine*, 62(5), 623-632.

- Chronic stress linked to abdominal fat accumulation

MINDFUL EATING AND BEHAVIOR CHANGE

1. Wansink, B. (2006). *Mindless Eating: Why We Eat More Than We Think*. New York: Bantam.

- Environmental and psychological factors affecting eating behavior

2. Robinson, E., et al. (2013). "Eating attentively: a systematic review and meta-analysis of the effect of food intake, memory, and awareness on eating." *American Journal of Clinical Nutrition*, 97(4), 728-742.

- Mindful eating reduces food intake

3. Prochaska, J. O., & DiClemente, C. C. (1983). "Stages and processes of self-change of smoking: toward an integrative model of change." *Journal of Consulting and Clinical Psychology*, 51(3), 390-395.

- Model for behavior change (applicable to dietary habits)

INFLAMMATION AND METABOLIC DISEASE

1. Hotamisligil, G. S. (2006). "Inflammation and metabolic disorders." *Nature*, 444(7121), 860-867.
   - Links chronic inflammation to obesity and metabolic disease
2. Calder, P. C., et al. (2011). "Dietary factors and low-grade inflammation in relation to overweight and obesity." *British Journal of Nutrition*, 106(S3), S5-S78.
   - How diet affects inflammation

LONGEVITY AND HEALTH SPAN

1. Fontana, L., & Partridge, L. (2015). "Promoting health and longevity through diet: from model organisms to humans." *Cell*, 161(1), 106-118.
   - Dietary strategies for longevity
2. Longo, V. D., et al. (2015). "Interventions to slow aging in humans: are we ready?" *Aging Cell*, 14(4), 497-510.
   - Evidence-based interventions for healthy aging

KEY BOOKS AND ADDITIONAL RESOURCES

1. Fung, J. (2016). *The Complete Guide to Fasting*. Las Vegas: Victory Belt Publishing.
2. Taubes, G. (2007). *Good Calories, Bad Calories*. New York: Alfred A. Knopf.
3. Teicholz, N. (2014). *The Big Fat Surprise*. New York: Simon & Schuster.
4. Perlmutter, D. (2013). *Grain Brain*. New York: Little, Brown and Company.

5.   Lustig, R. H. (2012). *Fat Chance: Beating the Odds Against Sugar, Processed Food, Obesity, and Disease.* New York: Hudson Street Press.

NOTE TO READERS

This reference list represents key scientific support for the concepts presented in this book. Science is constantly evolving, and readers are encouraged to stay informed about emerging research in metabolic health, nutrition, and longevity.

DID THIS BOOK HELP YOU?

If Fix Your Insulin has made a difference in your life — even a small one — I'd be incredibly grateful if you'd leave an honest review.

As an independent author, reviews are the single most important way new readers discover this book.

Your 30 seconds can help someone else escape the diet trap.

Leave your review at:
FixYourInsulin.com/review

Scan with your phone's camera or visit the link above.

Thank you for your support.

It means more than you know.

— Karl

9 7989 99 5015109